Contact Lens Design Tables

Contact Lens Design Tables

Tables for the determination of surface radii of curvature of hard contact lenses to give a required axial edge lift

Anthony Musset, DIC, PhD
Sequoia Air Ltd.
Janet Stone, FBCO, FAAO, DCLP
Senior Lecturer, The London Refraction Hospital

Butterworths
London Boston Sydney Wellington Durban Toronto

First published 1981

British Library Cataloguing in Publication Data

Musset, Anthony
Contact lens design tables.
1. Contact lenses – Handbooks, manuals, etc.
I. Title II. Stone, Janet
681′.423 QC372.6

ISBN 0-407-00219-7

Photoset by Butterworths Litho Preparation Department
Printed in England by Billing & Sons Ltd, Guildford and London

Contents

The Tables: these give Back Peripheral Optic Radii (Zonal Curvatures) for the following parameters (mm)

Introduction

These tables have been produced to help contact lens practitioners and manufacturers design co-axial multicurve lenses to give any desired axial edge lift. They are applicable to hard lenses and should prove useful now that new materials are available having better wetting properties and slight oxygen permeability, both of which permit greater flexibility in design. They can also be used for determining the specification of traditional polymethylmethacrylate lenses.

In order to follow the corneal contour and give peripheral corneal clearance, hard corneal contact lenses are usually made with the back peripheral zone having a different, flatter, curvature from that of the back central optic portion. There are other lens designs where the back surface consists of one aspheric curve or the peripheral curve is offset with respect to the central optic, but these are not common. In most lenses the back surface consists of two or more co-axial spherical curves. The axial edge lift of such a lens is defined by British Standards[1] as being the 'distance between a point on the back surface of a lens at a specified diameter, and the continuation of the back central optic portion, measured parallel to the axis of symmetry'. Generally the measurement is specified as being at the edge of the lens (*Figure 1.*).

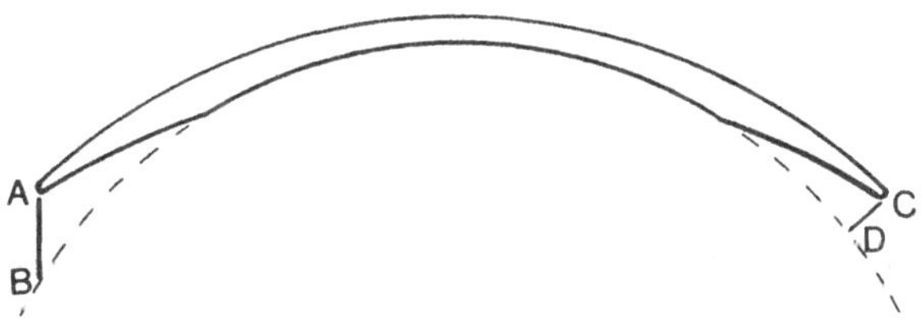

Figure 1 — AB is the axial edge lift and CD the radial edge lift of a corneal lens

It is important to realize that edge lift is a property of the lens itself. It is not the same as the edge clearance of the lens from the eye, although the two are obviously related. Axial rather than radial edge lift has been chosen since it is readily amenable to calculation from sagitta values; but there is a simple relation between the two (*see Note 1,* page *x*).

The back surface of a corneal lens rests on a layer of tears on the front surface of the cornea, which is itself aspheric, being approximately elliptical[2] in cross-section. It has been stated[3] that the peripheral zone of the lens must stand clear of the cornea for several reasons:

(1) To permit easy removal of the lens by enabling the lid margins to grip it.

(2) To allow the maintenance of adequate corneal metabolism by establishing under the periphery of the lens a reservoir of tears which can flow beneath the lens during eye movements, thereby providing oxygen to the cornea and removing metabolic waste products.

(3) To help centration of the lens on the cornea by providing a meniscus of tears which afford capillary attraction to offset gravitational effects which would otherwise cause the lens to drop.

(4) To prevent corneal damage occurring due to the edge digging into the corneal epithelium as the lens moves.

Consideration of these points in relation to the design of the back peripheral zone leads to the following conclusions.

(1) Where the axial edge lift is less than 0.08 mm, lenses generally become difficult to remove from the eye by manipulation of the eyelids, and a suction holder is usually required.

(2) The volume of tears fluid under the peripheral zone of a lens depends on a number of factors, one of them being the peripheral clearance of that lens from the cornea. Now on any given cornea the greater the axial edge lift of a lens the greater is its peripheral clearance. The volume also depends to some extent on the total width of the peripheral zone and on its shape, that is, the number of curves of which it is made up. Thus, as can be seen from *Figure 2,* a lens having a peripheral zone consisting of two curves contains a smaller volume of tears fluid than a single curve periphery, the axial edge lifts and the total peripheral zone widths being the same. Similarly, blending the transitions between peripheral zone curves increases the volume of tears under the periphery of the lens without affecting the axial edge lift; although the effect of blending the transition between the back central optic portion and the back peripheral zone will depend on the fit of the central portion. Where the central fit gives apical corneal clearance, blending this first transition will make the lens as a whole rest closer to the eye, thus reducing the volume of tears under the periphery.

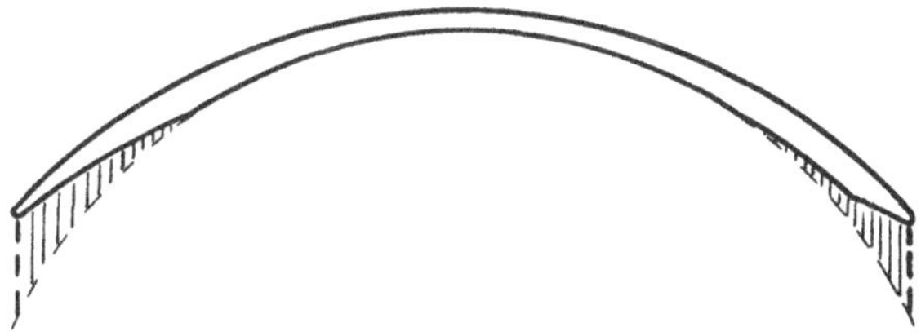

Figure 2 — The volume of tears under the peripheral zone on the right hand side, which has two curves, is seen to be less than that on the left hand side which has only one curve. On each side the axial edge lift and total peripheral zone width are the same

Where the central fit is in alignment or flatter than the cornea this does not apply. In fact, the volume of tears under the peripheral zone is increased. These points are illustrated in *Figures 3* and *4*. Thus, the choice of curves and the number of curves, as well as the amount of blending can influence the volume of the tears reservoir under the lens and this must be borne in mind when selecting peripheral curve radii.

Also to be considered here is the type of material from which the lens is made. If an oxygen-permeable material is used a smaller reservoir beneath the periphery of the lens may be acceptable, and the same applies, but to a slightly lesser extent, to materials with improved wettability compared to

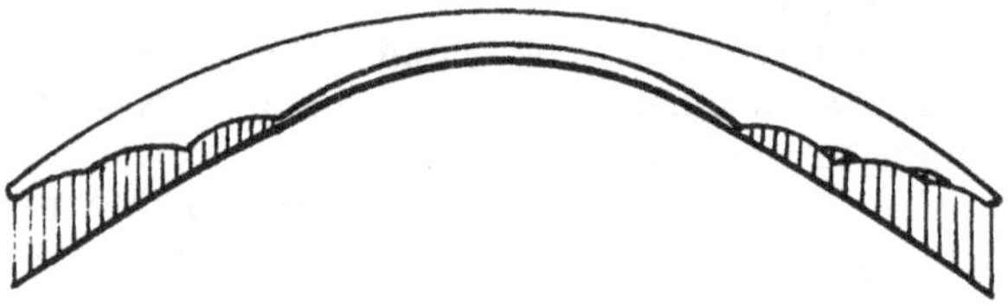

Figure 3 — This lens has three peripheral curves. On the right hand side the two transitions between these curves have been blended, and the increase in volume of tears under the peripheral zone, as compared to that on the left hand side, is apparent. The axial edge lift of the lens is unaffected by the blending, as is the edge clearance from the cornea

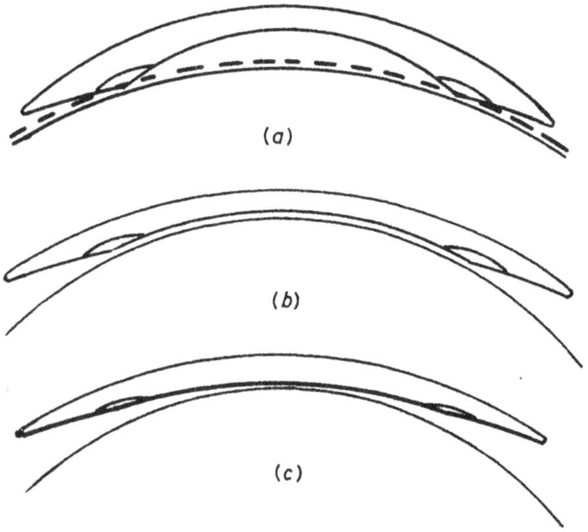

Figure 4— The effect of blending the transition between the back central optic portion and the back peripheral zone depends on the fit of the central portion. *(a)* If the central fit gives apical corneal clearance, the whole lens will rest closer to the cornea (then shown by the dashed line) and the volume of tears under both centre and periphery will be reduced. The axial edge lift of the lens is unaffected. *(b)* In an 'alignment' central fit, there will be a slight increase in the volume of tears under the peripheral zone. Again, the axial edge lift is unaffected. *(c)* With a flat central fit there is also a slight increase in the volume of tears under the peripheral zone, but the axial edge lift is not affected

polymethylmethacrylate. Alternatively, lenses of larger overall size and with larger back central optic portions may be acceptable in these newer materials, but maintaining similar axial edge lift.

(3) A lens which has a peripheral zone standing so much clear of the cornea as to introduce bubbles or even cause the tears meniscus to recede under the edge, defeats its own purpose (*Figure 5.*). Therefore, the use of lenses with too great an axial edge

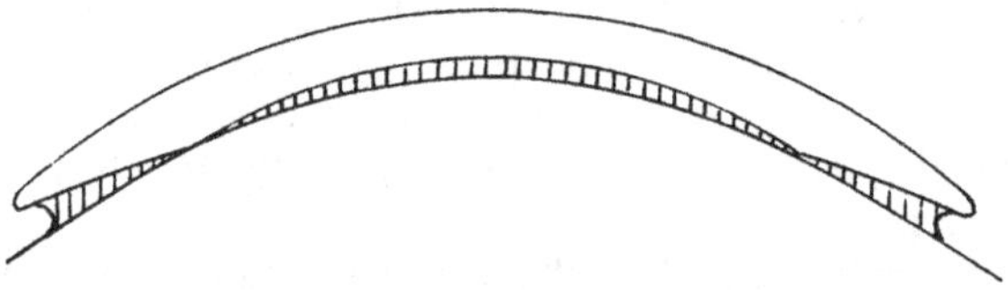

Figure 5 — Too great an axial edge lift gives too much peripheral corneal clearance at the edge of the lens, so that the tears meniscus recedes well inside the edge of the lens. Such lenses are uncomfortable, are easily dislodged on the eye, fall out easily, lead to '3 and 9 o'clock' corneal drying (accentuated if the lens has thick edges) and give rise to dimples in the corneal epithelium as a result of bubbles getting under the lens

lift is to be deprecated. Because corneas flatten peripherally at different rates, this aspect can best be studied by the use of trial lenses of known axial edge lift being observed on the eye using fluorescein and blue light. Observation with a slit lamp microscope using a circular aperture and magnification of *x*10 to *x*15 is useful, so that edge stand off during blinking and eye movements can be critically observed. Traditional methods of viewing the fluorescein picture with an ultraviolet lamp and central magnifier, whilst giving a good overall view of the total fluorescein pattern, do not give sufficient magnification to show the detail required.

(4) In order to prevent the lens edge digging into the corneal epithelium during blinking and eye movements the final peripheral curve on the back of the lens should be sufficiently flat to give a ski effect. Traditionally, a radius of 12.25 mm (obtained by using a tool of 1 inch diameter!) and a band width of 0.2 mm have been used, and these have been very successful in avoiding trauma. However, flatter curves may be needed on large lenses (overall sizes of 9.5 mm and more) especially on lenses with flat back central optic radii. Conversely, small lenses (overall sizes of 8.5 mm and less) especially with steep back central optic radii, rarely need quite such flat final peripheral radii, and curves down to 10.5 mm in radius are usually acceptable.

There are other factors to bear in mind when using these tables. Lenses having excessive peripheral corneal clearance, particularly if they also have thick edges, frequently give rise to 'three and nine o'clock' drying of the cornea, no matter how good is the wettability of the lens material.

The sharpness of a transition between two adjacent curves is related to the angle made at the junction between them (*Figure 6.*). The bigger the difference in radius between two adjacent co-axial curves the sharper this junction will be. But a 1mm

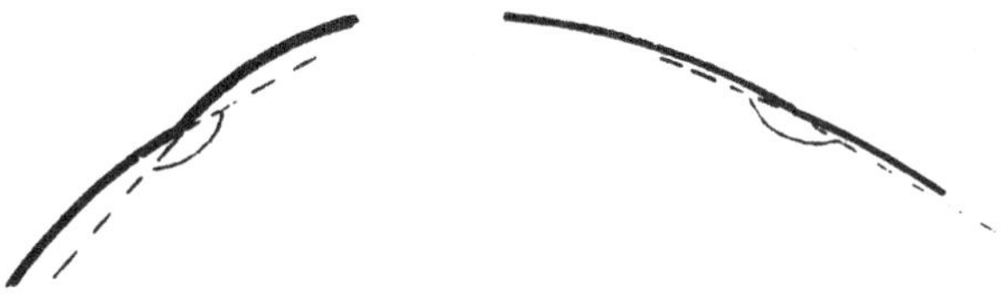

Figure 6 — The sharpness of a transition can be judged by the angle of junction between the two curves. On the left hand side, the transition between two relatively steep co-axial curves is shown, and on the right hand side between two flatter co-axial curves. On both sides the difference in radius between the two adjacent curves is the same. Although both junction angles are large, that on the right hand side is seen to be greater than that on the left

difference in radius between two steep curves, say radii of 7mm and 8mm, gives a much sharper junction than between two flat curves, say radii of 11mm and 12mm. Now because the lens is moving on the eye and is subject to pressure by the eyelids it is as well to avoid all sharp transitions, and, indeed, most laboratories blend them. However, the intrinsic design of the lens can avoid potentially sharp transitions by making small differences between adjacent radii for the inner back surface curves and using bigger differences for the outer curves.

Manufacturing accuracy and tolerances must be taken into account when designing lenses to give a specific axial edge lift. Bibby[4] has shown that for relatively steep peripheral radii (around 9.5mm) and large peripheral curve widths (around 0.9mm) an error in the radius has more effect on the edge lift than does an error in the width, whereas for relatively flat peripheral curve radii (around 13mm) and narrow widths (around 0.3mm) the converse is true.

To reiterate then, in selecting back surface radii the desirable features are as follows.

The first peripheral curve should be fairly close in radius to the BCOR to prevent a sharp transition, but progressing outwards the differences between adjacent radii may safely be increased.

The final peripheral curve should be flat enough to avoid digging into the cornea as the lens moves.

Very narrow zone widths should be avoided if manufacturers working to current tolerances are to produce sufficiently accurate lenses. This means that too many peripheral curves should be avoided. Small lenses (of overall size less than 8.6mm) are probably best manufactured in tricurve form, whereas lenses of average overall size (in the range 8.7mm to 9.5mm) may be tricurve or tetracurve, and for bigger lenses then pentacurve designs may be acceptable.

Experience with polymethylmethacrylate lenses for many years has led various practitioners[3, 5, 6, 7, 8] to quote desirable axial edge lift values at given overall sizes. Typical values are as follows:

Overall size (mm)	*Axial edge lifts (mm)*
8.2–8.7	0.11–0.13
8.8–9.2	0.13–0.16
9.3	0.16–0.20
10.1–12.5	0.18–0.50

For keratoconic eyes which must be fitted with lenses having fairly normal back peripheral radii but very steep central curvatures, axial edge lift values in excess of 0.25mm at an overall size of 9.0mm are not uncommon. Often with such very steep lenses, the need for such a large axial edge lift creates manufacturing difficulties. To minimize the problems likely to occur in manufacture it is recommended that such lenses are specified with as small an overall size and BCOD as possible.

Before dealing with the method of use of these tables, readers should understand how the total axial edge lift of the peripheral zone of the lens is made up. *Figure 7* shows a tricurve lens in which the axial

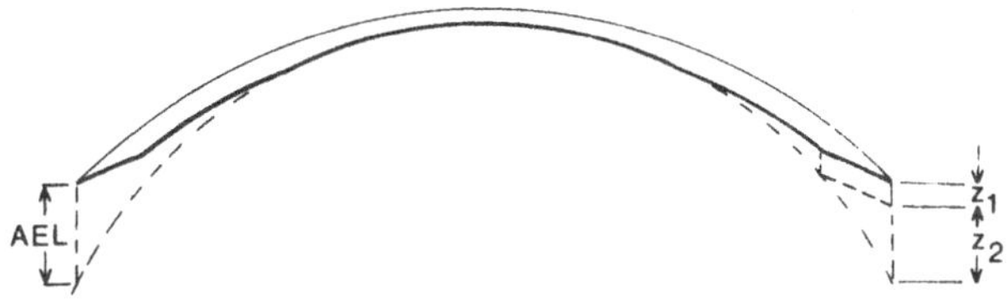

Figure 7 — In a tricurve lens, the axial edge lift, AEL, consists of two components, z_1 and z_2, contributed by the first and second peripheral curves respectively

edge lift has two components, z_1 and z_2. These are the contributions made by the first and second peripheral curves, respectively.

Generally speaking, for curves of similar widths the edge lift contribution should increase with each succeeding curve, as successively flatter peripheral radii are used. If the second peripheral curve contributed less to the axial edge lift than the first, and the two curves were of the same width, then the lens would be impossible to manufacture by normal techniques, as it would mean that the second peripheral curve was steeper than the first! Where the outermost peripheral curve is narrower than the others then this may not apply. The following section on the method of use of these tables illustrates the best approach to their use in lens design, and covers the selection of the various edge lift components to give satisfactory peripheral curve radii.

Note 1: Those who are used to working with radial edge lift will find the following formulae helpful.

$$z = \sqrt{(r + e)^2 - (d/2)^2} - \sqrt{r^2 - (d/2)^2}$$

$$e = \sqrt{r^2 + 2z\sqrt{r^2 - (d/2)^2 - r}}$$

z being the axial edge lift
e the radial edge lift
r the BCOR
d the OS

These formulae conveniently reduce to the approximate forms

$$z \doteqdot e(1 + d^2/8r^2)$$
$$e \doteqdot z(1 - d^2/8r^2)$$

Note 2: Throughout the Tables 'zonal curvatures' means back peripheral optic radii.

Method of Use of the Tables

There are seven tables in all. Tables I and II cover back central optic radii (BCOR) from 5.1mm to 6.9mm in 0.1mm steps. These two tables allow the design of lenses for all but the very steepest of keratoconic eyes, which are usually fitted with scleral lenses anyway. Both these tables cater for an inner diameter or back central optic diameter (BCOD) of 5.0mm. Because the number of keratoconic eyes is very few as compared to eyes of normal curvature, the peripheral zone widths (band widths) chosen for these tables are only two, namely 0.25mm in Table I and 0.5mm in Table II, going up to overall sizes (OS) of 10.0mm and 10.5mm in Tables I and II respectively.

The remaining tables (Tables III to VII) cater for the more usual BCOR values of 7.0–8.8mm, again in 0.1mm steps. Interpolation for BCOR values in 0.05mm steps is easily carried out. In these five tables BCOD values are either 6.0mm or 7.0mm, and peripheral zone widths are 0.2mm, 0.25mm, 0.3mm, 0.4mm and 0.5mm in each succeeding table, with OS values of 10.5–12.0mm.

Each table is arranged in fifteen sections, for edge lifts of 0.01–0.15mm in steps of 0.01mm. The sections themselves are divided up into a series of double lines, the upper of the two lines giving the edge lift component and the inner and outer diameters to which it applies. The lower of the two lines gives the back peripheral radii (zonal curvatures as they are called in these tables) necessary to achieve the stated edge lift component for the range of BCOR values used in that particular table. All the back peripheral radii are rounded to the nearest 0.05mm, and superfluous zeros and decimal points have been omitted. The mm abbreviations for millimetres have also been omitted throughout the tables.

Looking at the first section of Table I, it is seen to apply to edge lifts of 0.01 and consists of ten double lines. The uppermost pair of these, besides stating the edge lift component of 0.01 states the inner and outer optic diameters as being 5.0–5.5, that is, a zone width of 0.25. The zonal curvatures follow in the lower of the pair of lines, which thus show the back peripheral radii which will give an axial edge lift component of 0.01 for BCOR values ranging from 5.1 in 0.1 steps to 6.9. Nineteen values are therefore shown in this lower line.

For example, if a lens is needed having BCOR 5.1, BCOD 5.0 and with the first band of the peripheral zone 0.25 wide (outer diameter of this band is 5.5), then for this peripheral band to contribute 0.01 to the axial edge lift, the desired back peripheral radius is the first value on the left, which is 5.35.

If, however, the BCOR needed is 5.8, rather than 5.1, then the eighth value along from the left must be taken, which is seen to be 6.2.

Now an example of the design of the back surface of a complete lens will be considered. It is recommended that readers check the values in the tables as they work through the example.

Taking more usual parameters than those just illustrated, consider the design of a lens having a BCOR of 7.8, BCOD of 7.0 and OS of 9.0. The axial edge lift required is 0.14.

First a decision must be made on the number of peripheral curves required and their widths. As it is common to have lenses of this OS and BCOD made in tetracurve form, three peripheral curves will be used in this illustration. As a flat final (or third) peripheral curve over a narrow band is ideal, a width of 0.2 will be allocated for this curve, giving it inner and outer diameters of 8.6 and 9.0. The remainder of the peripheral zone may as well have curves of equal width, making them 0.4 wide, with inner and outer diameters of the first peripheral curve being 7.0 and 7.8, and of the second peripheral curve 7.8 and 8.6.

Writing this in British Standard recommended form, the lens specification so far determined is: C4/7.80:7.0/? :7.8/? :8.6/? :9.0

There are a number of ways in which these three peripheral curves can contribute to the total edge lift of 0.14. Bearing in mind the optimum type of design, discussed earlier, a first peripheral curve fairly close to the BCOR is desirable to prevent too sharp a transition. Table VI, for peripheral curve widths of 0.4, must be used to select this curve. This table covers BCOR values from 7.0 to 8.8, so that for a BCOR of 7.8 the ninth value from the left hand side must be taken in any line of figures, since the BCOR values progress in steps of 0.1. Looking at the 0.01 edge lift components for optic diameters of 7.0–7.8 gives a peripheral curve of 8.1. The 0.02 edge lift component gives 8.4 and the 0.03 edge lift gives 8.8.

Of these, the 0.02 edge lift component giving a first peripheral curve of 8.4 is probably the most desirable, but a 0.03 component giving a radius of 8.8 is also acceptable.

Next, take the third or final peripheral curve. This requires the use of Table III for zone widths of 0.2. The optic diameters involved are 8.6 and 9.0. Looking always at the ninth zonal curvature value from the left, for various edge lift components and the optic diameters of 8.6–9.0, it will be seen that the following applies:

Edge lift (mm)	*Zonal curvature (mm)*
0.04	10.1
0.05	11.05
0.06	12.3
0.07	13.9

From experience it is known that the values 11.05, 12.3 or 13.9 would all be acceptable, but probably 12.3 is the best value giving an edge lift component of 0.06.

Thus, with a first peripheral curve of 8.4 contributing 0.02 to the edge lift, and a final peripheral curve of 12.3 contributing a further 0.06, to give a total axial edge lift of 0.14, the remaining peripheral curve must contribute another 0.06. To select this Table VI must be consulted again for optic diameters of 7.8–8.6. At an edge lift of 0.06 the ninth value from the left is 9.65 making this the radius of the second peripheral curve. The lens specification is thus:

C4/7.80:7.0/8.40:7.8/9.65:8.6/12.3:9.0 (1)

Had 11.05 been chosen for the final peripheral curve (contributing 0.05 to the edge lift), then the second peripheral curve could have remained as 9.65 (contributing 0.06 to the edge lift), but the first peripheral curve would then have to contribute 0.03 to the edge lift, which makes the radius 8.8, and, as stated above, this is acceptable.

The lens specification then becomes:

C4/7.80:7.0/8.80:7.8/9.65:8.6/11.05:9.0 (2)

Alternatively, the first peripheral curve could be kept at 8.4 as in (1) above, and the second peripheral curve altered to give an edge lift component of 0.07. Consulting Table VI again for optic diameters of 7.8–8.6 and for an edge lift component of 0.07 gives a value of 10.1 (ninth from the left).

This results in the lens:

C4/7.80:7.0/8.4:7.8/10.1:8.6/11.05:9.0 (3)

Lenses (1), (2) and (3) all have an axial edge lift of 0.14. By simple interpolation other values again could be chosen. For example, a final peripheral curve of 11.675 (midway between 11.05 and 12.3) would give an edge lift component of 0.055 (not given directly in Table III). The second peripheral curve could then contribute 0.065 to the edge lift, making its radius 9.875 (midway between 9.65 and 10.1). With these figures rounded to two places of decimals, the lens becomes:

C4/7.80:7.0/8.40:7.8/9.9:8.6/11.70:9.0 (4)

The final choice would probably be lenses (1) or (4) as the progression of curves in both lenses is such as to minimize the sharpness of the transitions between adjacent curves. Lens (1) is therefore the lens of choice, unless the user is prepared to interpolate in the tables.

The above example of choosing a lens specification to give a required axial edge lift, brings out one further point. This is that quite large changes in radius are needed to make a 0.01 edge lift component change on the narrow final peripheral curve. Thus, it is likely to have very little effect on the edge lift or the peripheral corneal clearance if these final peripheral curve values are rounded to a figure corresponding to the manufacturer's usual range of tools. For example, 12.3 could be written as 12.25 without seriously upsetting the specification, and 11.7 could be 11.75. The method of manufacture would influence this, as only a few manufacturers lathe-cut their peripheral curves to any desired radius, whereas most use diamond-impregnated brass radius tools, and they may only have these available in 0.25 steps for radii flatter than 10.0.

In parts of the tables it will be seen that the letters NE replace the usual values for zonal curvature. This occurs where such values do not exist.

It will also be seen that many very flat radii (for example, 59.1) have been included. They allow users to assess the feasibility of manufacturing lenses of some desired design. In fact, few manufacturers will normally make radii flatter than 17.5.

It is hoped that these tables will prove useful to both practitioners and manufacturers by permitting easy determination of the back surface specification of both simple and more sophisticated hard lens designs. Other aspects of corneal lens design are well covered elsewhere [9, 10, 11] and these sources should be consulted for a fuller understanding of the subject.

References

1 BRITISH STANDARD 3521 (1979). *Glossary of Terms Relating to Ophthalmic Lenses and Spectacle Frames*. Part 3: 'Glossary of terms relating to contact lenses. London: British Standards Institution

2 SENFF, R. (1846). Quoted by Helmholtz, H. V. (1909). *Handbuch der Physiologischen Optik*. English translation edited by Southall, J. P. C. (1962). *Treatise on Physiological Optics*. London: Dover Publications

3 STONE, J. (1975). 'Corneal lenses with constant axial edge lift.' *Ophthal. Optician* **15,** 1,818–824

4 BIBBY, M. (1979). 'Factors affecting peripheral curve design.' *Am. J. Optom.* **56,** 1, 2–9, and 'Factors affecting peripheral curve design. Part II: Specifying for reproducible performance.' *Am. J. Optom.* **56,** 10, 618–627

5 RABBETTS, R. B. (1976). 'Large corneal lenses with constant axial edge lift.' *Ophthal Optician.* **16,** 236, 239

6 ATKINSON, T. C. O. (1980). 'The return of hard times, Part II, or the changing "value" of edge lift.' *J. Br. Contact Lens Ass.* **3,** 3, 105–112

7 MARRIOTT, P. J. (1978). Personal communication

8 FORD, M. W. (1979). Personal communication

9 STONE, J. AND PHILLIPS, A. J. (1980–1981). *Contact Lenses, Vols 1 and 2, 2nd ed.* London: Butterworths

10 CREIGHTON, C. P. (1964). *Contact Lenses Fabrication Tables.* New York: Creighton

11 STONE, J. (1981). 'Designing hard lenses in the 1980s'. Awaiting publication in *J. Br. Contact Lens Ass.*

TABLE I Back Peripheral Optic Radii (Zonal Curvatures) for the following:
BCOR 5.1 to 6.9 in 0.1 steps
Zone Width 0.25 Zone Inner Diameters 5.0 to 9.5 in 0.5 steps
Axial Edge Lift Components 0.01 to 0.15 in 0.01 steps

FOR EDGE LIFT 0.01 , OPTIC DIAMETERS 5 - 5.5 , ZONAL CURVATURES ARE

5.35 5.5 5.6 5.7 5.85 5.95 6.1 6.2 6.3 6.45 6.55 6.7 6.8 6.9 7.05 7.15 7.3 7.4 7.55

FOR EDGE LIFT 0.01 , OPTIC DIAMETERS 5.5 - 6 , ZONAL CURVATURES ARE

5.3 5.45 5.55 5.65 5.8 5.9 6 6.15 6.25 6.35 6.5 6.6 6.7 6.85 6.95 7.1 7.2 7.35 7.45

FOR EDGE LIFT 0.01 , OPTIC DIAMETERS 6 - 6.5 , ZONAL CURVATURES ARE

5.25 5.4 5.5 5.6 5.75 5.85 5.95 6.1 6.2 6.3 6.45 6.55 6.65 6.8 6.9 7 7.15 7.25 7.35

FOR EDGE LIFT 0.01 , OPTIC DIAMETERS 6.5 - 7 , ZONAL CURVATURES ARE

5.25 5.35 5.45 5.55 5.7 5.8 5.9 6.05 6.15 6.25 6.35 6.5 6.6 6.7 6.85 6.95 7.05 7.2 7.3

FOR EDGE LIFT 0.01 , OPTIC DIAMETERS 7 - 7.5 , ZONAL CURVATURES ARE

5.2 5.3 5.45 5.55 5.65 5.75 5.85 6 6.1 6.2 6.35 6.45 6.55 6.65 6.8 6.9 7 7.15 7.25

FOR EDGE LIFT 0.01 , OPTIC DIAMETERS 7.5 - 8 , ZONAL CURVATURES ARE

5.2 5.3 5.4 5.5 5.6 5.75 5.85 5.95 6.05 6.15 6.3 6.4 6.5 6.65 6.75 6.85 6.95 7.1 7.2

FOR EDGE LIFT 0.01 , OPTIC DIAMETERS 8 - 8.5 , ZONAL CURVATURES ARE

5.15 5.25 5.35 5.5 5.6 5.7 5.8 5.9 6.05 6.15 6.25 6.35 6.5 6.6 6.7 6.8 6.95 7.05 7.15

FOR EDGE LIFT 0.01 , OPTIC DIAMETERS 8.5 - 9 , ZONAL CURVATURES ARE

5.15 5.25 5.35 5.45 5.55 5.65 5.8 5.9 6 6.1 6.2 6.35 6.45 6.55 6.65 6.8 6.9 7 7.1

FOR EDGE LIFT 0.01 , OPTIC DIAMETERS 9 - 9.5 , ZONAL CURVATURES ARE

5.1 5.2 5.35 5.45 5.55 5.65 5.75 5.85 5.95 6.1 6.2 6.3 6.4 6.5 6.65 6.75 6.85 6.95 7.1

FOR EDGE LIFT 0.01 , OPTIC DIAMETERS 9.5 - 10 , ZONAL CURVATURES ARE

5.1 5.2 5.3 5.4 5.5 5.65 5.75 5.85 5.95 6.05 6.15 6.3 6.4 6.5 6.6 6.7 6.8 6.95 7.05

FOR EDGE LIFT 0.02 , OPTIC DIAMETERS 5 - 5.5 , ZONAL CURVATURES ARE

5.7 5.8 5.95 6.1 6.25 6.4 6.55 6.7 6.8 6.95 7.1 7.25 7.4 7.55 7.7 7.9 8.05 8.2 8.35

FOR EDGE LIFT 0.02 , OPTIC DIAMETERS 5.5 - 6 , ZONAL CURVATURES ARE

5.55 5.7 5.85 5.95 6.1 6.25 6.4 6.5 6.65 6.8 6.95 7.1 7.25 7.4 7.55 7.7 7.8 7.95 8.1

FOR EDGE LIFT 0.02 , OPTIC DIAMETERS 6 - 6.5 , ZONAL CURVATURES ARE

5.45 5.6 5.75 5.85 6 6.15 6.25 6.4 6.55 6.65 6.8 6.95 7.1 7.25 7.35 7.5 7.65 7.8 7.95

FOR EDGE LIFT 0.02 , OPTIC DIAMETERS 6.5 - 7 , ZONAL CURVATURES ARE

5.4 5.5 5.65 5.75 5.9 6.05 6.15 6.3 6.4 6.55 6.7 6.8 6.95 7.1 7.25 7.35 7.5 7.65 7.8

FOR EDGE LIFT 0.02 , OPTIC DIAMETERS 7 - 7.5 , ZONAL CURVATURES ARE

5.3 5.45 5.55 5.7 5.8 5.95 6.05 6.2 6.35 6.45 6.6 6.7 6.85 7 7.1 7.25 7.4 7.5 7.65

FOR EDGE LIFT 0.02 , OPTIC DIAMETERS 7.5 - 8 , ZONAL CURVATURES ARE

5.25 5.4 5.5 5.6 5.75 5.85 6 6.1 6.25 6.35 6.5 6.65 6.75 6.9 7 7.15 7.3 7.4 7.55

FOR EDGE LIFT 0.02 , OPTIC DIAMETERS 8 - 8.5 , ZONAL CURVATURES ARE

5.2 5.35 5.45 5.55 5.7 5.8 5.95 6.05 6.15 6.3 6.4 6.55 6.65 6.8 6.95 7.05 7.2 7.3 7.45

FOR EDGE LIFT 0.02 , OPTIC DIAMETERS 8.5 - 9 , ZONAL CURVATURES ARE

5.15 5.3 5.4 5.5 5.65 5.75 5.85 6 6.1 6.25 6.35 6.5 6.6 6.7 6.85 6.95 7.1 7.25 7.35

FOR EDGE LIFT 0.02 , OPTIC DIAMETERS 9 - 9.5 , ZONAL CURVATURES ARE

5.15 5.25 5.35 5.45 5.6 5.7 5.8 5.95 6.05 6.15 6.3 6.4 6.55 6.65 6.8 6.9 7.05 7.15 7.3

FOR EDGE LIFT 0.02 , OPTIC DIAMETERS 9.5 - 10 , ZONAL CURVATURES ARE

5.1 5.2 5.35 5.45 5.55 5.65 5.8 5.9 6 6.15 6.25 6.35 6.5 6.6 6.7 6.85 6.95 7.1 7.2

```
FOR EDGE LIFT   0.03 ,   OPTIC DIAMETERS   5 - 5.5 ,   ZONAL CURVATURES ARE
 6.05 6.25 6.4 6.55 6.75 6.9 7.1 7.25 7.45 7.65 7.8 8 8.2 8.4 8.6 8.75 8.95 9.2 9.4

FOR EDGE LIFT   0.03 ,   OPTIC DIAMETERS   5.5 - 6 ,   ZONAL CURVATURES ARE
 5.85 6 6.2 6.35 6.5 6.65 6.85 7 7.15 7.35 7.5 7.7 7.85 8.05 8.2 8.4 8.6 8.8 8.95

FOR EDGE LIFT   0.03 ,   OPTIC DIAMETERS   6 - 6.5 ,   ZONAL CURVATURES ARE
 5.7 5.85 6 6.15 6.3 6.45 6.6 6.8 6.95 7.1 7.25 7.45 7.6 7.75 7.95 8.1 8.3 8.45 8.65

FOR EDGE LIFT   0.03 ,   OPTIC DIAMETERS   6.5 - 7 ,   ZONAL CURVATURES ARE
 5.55 5.7 5.85 6 6.15 6.3 6.45 6.6 6.75 6.9 7.05 7.2 7.4 7.55 7.7 7.85 8.05 8.2 8.35

FOR EDGE LIFT   0.03 ,   OPTIC DIAMETERS   7 - 7.5 ,   ZONAL CURVATURES ARE
 5.45 5.6 5.75 5.85 6 6.15 6.3 6.45 6.6 6.75 6.9 7.05 7.2 7.35 7.5 7.65 7.8 8 8.15

FOR EDGE LIFT   0.03 ,   OPTIC DIAMETERS   7.5 - 8 ,   ZONAL CURVATURES ARE
 5.35 5.5 5.6 5.75 5.9 6.05 6.15 6.3 6.45 6.6 6.75 6.9 7.05 7.2 7.35 7.5 7.65 7.8 7.95

FOR EDGE LIFT   0.03 ,   OPTIC DIAMETERS   8 - 8.5 ,   ZONAL CURVATURES ARE
 5.25 5.4 5.55 5.65 5.8 5.95 6.05 6.2 6.35 6.45 6.6 6.75 6.9 7.05 7.2 7.35 7.5 7.65 7.75

FOR EDGE LIFT   0.03 ,   OPTIC DIAMETERS   8.5 - 9 ,   ZONAL CURVATURES ARE
 5.2 5.35 5.45 5.6 5.7 5.85 5.95 6.1 6.25 6.35 6.5 6.65 6.8 6.9 7.05 7.2 7.35 7.5 7.65

FOR EDGE LIFT   0.03 ,   OPTIC DIAMETERS   9 - 9.5 ,   ZONAL CURVATURES ARE
 5.15 5.25 5.4 5.5 5.65 5.75 5.9 6 6.15 6.25 6.4 6.55 6.65 6.8 6.95 7.1 7.2 7.35 7.5

FOR EDGE LIFT   0.03 ,   OPTIC DIAMETERS   9.5 - 10 ,   ZONAL CURVATURES ARE
 5.1 5.25 5.35 5.45 5.6 5.7 5.8 5.95 6.05 6.2 6.3 6.45 6.6 6.7 6.85 7 7.1 7.25 7.4
```

FOR EDGE LIFT 0.04 , OPTIC DIAMETERS 5 - 5.5 , ZONAL CURVATURES ARE

6.5 6.7 6.9 7.1 7.35 7.55 7.75 8 8.2 8.45 8.7 8.95 9.2 9.45 9.7 9.95 10.2 10.5 10.75

FOR EDGE LIFT 0.04 , OPTIC DIAMETERS 5.5 - 6 , ZONAL CURVATURES ARE

6.2 6.4 6.6 6.75 6.95 7.15 7.35 7.55 7.75 8 8.2 8.4 8.65 8.85 9.1 9.35 9.55 9.8 10.05

FOR EDGE LIFT 0.04 , OPTIC DIAMETERS 6 - 6.5 , ZONAL CURVATURES ARE

5.95 6.15 6.3 6.5 6.65 6.85 7.05 7.2 7.4 7.6 7.8 8 8.2 8.4 8.65 8.85 9.05 9.3 9.5

FOR EDGE LIFT 0.04 , OPTIC DIAMETERS 6.5 - 7 , ZONAL CURVATURES ARE

5.75 5.9 6.1 6.25 6.4 6.6 6.75 6.95 7.15 7.3 7.5 7.7 7.85 8.05 8.25 8.45 8.65 8.85 9.05

FOR EDGE LIFT 0.04 , OPTIC DIAMETERS 7 - 7.5 , ZONAL CURVATURES ARE

5.6 5.75 5.9 6.05 6.2 6.4 6.55 6.7 6.9 7.05 7.25 7.4 7.6 7.75 7.95 8.15 8.35 8.5 8.7

FOR EDGE LIFT 0.04 , OPTIC DIAMETERS 7.5 - 8 , ZONAL CURVATURES ARE

5.45 5.6 5.75 5.9 6.05 6.2 6.35 6.5 6.7 6.85 7 7.2 7.35 7.5 7.7 7.85 8.05 8.25 8.4

FOR EDGE LIFT 0.04 , OPTIC DIAMETERS 8 - 8.5 , ZONAL CURVATURES ARE

5.35 5.5 5.6 5.75 5.9 6.05 6.2 6.35 6.5 6.65 6.85 7 7.15 7.3 7.5 7.65 7.8 8 8.15

FOR EDGE LIFT 0.04 , OPTIC DIAMETERS 8.5 - 9 , ZONAL CURVATURES ARE

5.25 5.4 5.5 5.65 5.8 5.95 6.05 6.2 6.35 6.5 6.65 6.8 6.95 7.15 7.3 7.45 7.6 7.8 7.95

FOR EDGE LIFT 0.04 , OPTIC DIAMETERS 9 - 9.5 , ZONAL CURVATURES ARE

5.15 5.3 5.45 5.55 5.7 5.8 5.95 6.1 6.25 6.4 6.55 6.7 6.8 6.95 7.15 7.3 7.45 7.6 7.75

FOR EDGE LIFT 0.04 , OPTIC DIAMETERS 9.5 - 10 , ZONAL CURVATURES ARE

5.1 5.25 5.35 5.5 5.6 5.75 5.85 6 6.15 6.25 6.4 6.55 6.7 6.85 7 7.15 7.3 7.45 7.6

FOR EDGE LIFT 0.05 , OPTIC DIAMETERS 5 - 5.5 , ZONAL CURVATURES ARE

7.05 7.3 7.55 7.8 8.1 8.35 8.65 8.95 9.2 9.55 9.85 10.15 10.5 10.85 11.2 11.55 11.9 12.3 12.7

FOR EDGE LIFT 0.05 , OPTIC DIAMETERS 5.5 - 6 , ZONAL CURVATURES ARE

6.6 6.85 7.05 7.3 7.55 7.75 8 8.25 8.55 8.8 9.05 9.35 9.6 9.9 10.2 10.5 10.85 11.15 11.5

FOR EDGE LIFT 0.05 , OPTIC DIAMETERS 6 - 6.5 , ZONAL CURVATURES ARE

6.25 6.45 6.65 6.9 7.1 7.3 7.55 7.75 8 8.25 8.45 8.7 9 9.25 9.5 9.75 10.05 10.35 10.6

FOR EDGE LIFT 0.05 , OPTIC DIAMETERS 6.5 - 7 , ZONAL CURVATURES ARE

6 6.15 6.35 6.55 6.75 6.95 7.15 7.35 7.6 7.8 8 8.25 8.45 8.7 8.95 9.2 9.45 9.7 9.95

FOR EDGE LIFT 0.05 , OPTIC DIAMETERS 7 - 7.5 , ZONAL CURVATURES ARE

5.75 5.95 6.1 6.3 6.45 6.65 6.85 7.05 7.25 7.45 7.65 7.85 8.05 8.25 8.5 8.7 8.95 9.15 9.4

FOR EDGE LIFT 0.05 , OPTIC DIAMETERS 7.5 - 8 , ZONAL CURVATURES ARE

5.55 5.75 5.9 6.05 6.25 6.4 6.6 6.75 6.95 7.15 7.35 7.5 7.7 7.9 8.1 8.35 8.55 8.75 8.95

FOR EDGE LIFT 0.05 , OPTIC DIAMETERS 8 - 8.5 , ZONAL CURVATURES ARE

5.4 5.55 5.7 5.9 6.05 6.2 6.35 6.55 6.7 6.9 7.05 7.25 7.45 7.6 7.8 8 8.2 8.4 8.6

FOR EDGE LIFT 0.05 , OPTIC DIAMETERS 8.5 - 9 , ZONAL CURVATURES ARE

5.3 5.45 5.6 5.75 5.9 6.05 6.2 6.35 6.5 6.7 6.85 7 7.2 7.35 7.55 7.75 7.9 8.1 8.3

FOR EDGE LIFT 0.05 , OPTIC DIAMETERS 9 - 9.5 , ZONAL CURVATURES ARE

5.2 5.35 5.45 5.6 5.75 5.9 6.05 6.2 6.35 6.5 6.65 6.85 7 7.15 7.35 7.5 7.7 7.85 8.05

FOR EDGE LIFT 0.05 , OPTIC DIAMETERS 9.5 - 10 , ZONAL CURVATURES ARE

5.1 5.25 5.35 5.5 5.65 5.8 5.9 6.05 6.2 6.35 6.5 6.65 6.8 7 7.15 7.3 7.45 7.65 7.8

```
FOR EDGE LIFT   6.00000E-2 ,   OPTIC DIAMETERS   5 - 5.5 ,   ZONAL CURVATURES ARE
 7.75  8.05  8.35  8.7  9.05  9.4  9.75  10.15  10.55  10.95  11.4  11.85  12.3  12.8  13.3  13.8  14.35  14.95  15.55

FOR EDGE LIFT   6.00000E-2 ,   OPTIC DIAMETERS   5.5 - 6 ,   ZONAL CURVATURES ARE
 7.1  7.35  7.65  7.95  8.2  8.5  8.85  9.15  9.5  9.8  10.2  10.55  10.9  11.3  11.7  12.15  12.55  13  13.45

FOR EDGE LIFT   6.00000E-2 ,   OPTIC DIAMETERS   6 - 6.5 ,   ZONAL CURVATURES ARE
 6.6  6.85  7.1  7.35  7.6  7.85  8.15  8.4  8.7  9  9.3  9.6  9.95  10.25  10.6  10.95  11.3  11.7  12.05

FOR EDGE LIFT   6.00000E-2 ,   OPTIC DIAMETERS   6.5 - 7 ,   ZONAL CURVATURES ARE
 6.25  6.45  6.65  6.9  7.15  7.35  7.6  7.85  8.1  8.35  8.65  8.9  9.2  9.5  9.8  10.1  10.4  10.7  11.05

FOR EDGE LIFT   6.00000E-2 ,   OPTIC DIAMETERS   7 - 7.5 ,   ZONAL CURVATURES ARE
 5.95  6.15  6.35  6.55  6.75  6.95  7.2  7.4  7.65  7.9  8.1  8.35  8.6  8.85  9.15  9.4  9.7  9.95  10.25

FOR EDGE LIFT   6.00000E-2 ,   OPTIC DIAMETERS   7.5 - 8 ,   ZONAL CURVATURES ARE
 5.7  5.85  6.05  6.25  6.45  6.65  6.85  7.05  7.25  7.45  7.7  7.9  8.15  8.4  8.65  8.85  9.1  9.4  9.65

FOR EDGE LIFT   6.00000E-2 ,   OPTIC DIAMETERS   8 - 8.5 ,   ZONAL CURVATURES ARE
 5.5  5.65  5.85  6  6.2  6.35  6.55  6.75  6.95  7.15  7.35  7.55  7.75  8  8.2  8.45  8.65  8.9  9.15

FOR EDGE LIFT   6.00000E-2 ,   OPTIC DIAMETERS   8.5 - 9 ,   ZONAL CURVATURES ARE
 5.35  5.5  5.65  5.8  6  6.15  6.3  6.5  6.7  6.85  7.05  7.25  7.45  7.65  7.85  8.05  8.3  8.5  8.7

FOR EDGE LIFT   6.00000E-2 ,   OPTIC DIAMETERS   9 - 9.5 ,   ZONAL CURVATURES ARE
 5.2  5.35  5.5  5.65  5.8  5.95  6.15  6.3  6.45  6.65  6.8  7  7.2  7.35  7.55  7.75  7.95  8.15  8.35

FOR EDGE LIFT   6.00000E-2 ,   OPTIC DIAMETERS   9.5 - 10 ,   ZONAL CURVATURES ARE
 5.15  5.25  5.4  5.55  5.65  5.8  5.95  6.15  6.3  6.45  6.6  6.8  6.95  7.15  7.3  7.5  7.7  7.85  8.05
```

```
FOR EDGE LIFT   0.07 ,   OPTIC DIAMETERS   5 - 5.5 ,   ZONAL CURVATURES ARE
8.6  9  9.4  9.85  10.3  10.8  11.3  11.8  12.4  12.95  13.6  14.25  14.95  15.7  16.45  17.3  18.2  19.15  20.15

FOR EDGE LIFT   0.07 ,   OPTIC DIAMETERS   5.5 - 6 ,   ZONAL CURVATURES ARE
7.7  8  8.35  8.7  9.1  9.45  9.85  10.3  10.75  11.2  11.65  12.15  12.65  13.2  13.8  14.4  15  15.65  16.35

FOR EDGE LIFT   0.07 ,   OPTIC DIAMETERS   6 - 6.5 ,   ZONAL CURVATURES ARE
7.05  7.3  7.6  7.9  8.2  8.55  8.9  9.25  9.6  9.95  10.35  10.75  11.15  11.6  12.05  12.5  13  13.5  14.05

FOR EDGE LIFT   0.07 ,   OPTIC DIAMETERS   6.5 - 7 ,   ZONAL CURVATURES ARE
6.55  6.8  7.05  7.3  7.6  7.85  8.15  8.45  8.75  9.1  9.4  9.75  10.1  10.45  10.85  11.25  11.65  12.05  12.5

FOR EDGE LIFT   0.07 ,   OPTIC DIAMETERS   7 - 7.5 ,   ZONAL CURVATURES ARE
6.15  6.35  6.6  6.85  7.05  7.3  7.6  7.85  8.1  8.4  8.7  9  9.3  9.6  9.95  10.25  10.6  10.95  11.35

FOR EDGE LIFT   0.07 ,   OPTIC DIAMETERS   7.5 - 8 ,   ZONAL CURVATURES ARE
5.85  6.05  6.25  6.45  6.65  6.9  7.15  7.35  7.6  7.85  8.1  8.4  8.65  8.95  9.25  9.5  9.85  10.15  10.45

FOR EDGE LIFT   0.07 ,   OPTIC DIAMETERS   8 - 8.5 ,   ZONAL CURVATURES ARE
5.6  5.75  5.95  6.15  6.35  6.55  6.75  7  7.2  7.45  7.65  7.9  8.15  8.4  8.65  8.95  9.2  9.5  9.75

FOR EDGE LIFT   0.07 ,   OPTIC DIAMETERS   8.5 - 9 ,   ZONAL CURVATURES ARE
5.4  5.55  5.7  5.9  6.1  6.25  6.45  6.65  6.85  7.1  7.3  7.5  7.75  7.95  8.2  8.45  8.7  8.95  9.2

FOR EDGE LIFT   0.07 ,   OPTIC DIAMETERS   9 - 9.5 ,   ZONAL CURVATURES ARE
5.25  5.4  5.55  5.7  5.9  6.05  6.25  6.4  6.6  6.8  7  7.2  7.4  7.6  7.8  8.05  8.25  8.5  8.75

FOR EDGE LIFT   0.07 ,   OPTIC DIAMETERS   9.5 - 10 ,   ZONAL CURVATURES ARE
5.15  5.25  5.4  5.55  5.7  5.85  6.05  6.2  6.35  6.55  6.75  6.9  7.1  7.3  7.5  7.7  7.9  8.15  8.35
```

```
FOR EDGE LIFT   0.08 ,   OPTIC DIAMETERS   5 - 5.5 ,   ZONAL CURVATURES ARE
 9.7  10.25  10.8  11.4  12.05  12.7  13.45  14.25  15.05  15.95  16.95  18  19.15  20.4  21.75  23.25  24.9  26.75  28.8

FOR EDGE LIFT   0.08 ,   OPTIC DIAMETERS   5.5 - 6 ,   ZONAL CURVATURES ARE
 8.45  8.85  9.25  9.75  10.2  10.7  11.25  11.8  12.4  13.05  13.7  14.4  15.15  16  16.85  17.75  18.75  19.8  20.95

FOR EDGE LIFT   0.08 ,   OPTIC DIAMETERS   6 - 6.5 ,   ZONAL CURVATURES ARE
 7.55  7.85  8.25  8.6  9  9.4  9.8  10.25  10.7  11.2  11.7  12.25  12.8  13.4  14.05  14.7  15.4  16.1  16.9

FOR EDGE LIFT   0.08 ,   OPTIC DIAMETERS   6.5 - 7 ,   ZONAL CURVATURES ARE
 6.9  7.15  7.45  7.8  8.1  8.45  8.8  9.15  9.55  9.95  10.35  10.8  11.25  11.7  12.2  12.7  13.25  13.8  14.4

FOR EDGE LIFT   0.08 ,   OPTIC DIAMETERS   7 - 7.5 ,   ZONAL CURVATURES ARE
 6.35  6.65  6.9  7.15  7.45  7.75  8.05  8.35  8.7  9.05  9.4  9.75  10.1  10.5  10.9  11.35  11.8  12.25  12.7

FOR EDGE LIFT   0.08 ,   OPTIC DIAMETERS   7.5 - 8 ,   ZONAL CURVATURES ARE
 6  6.2  6.45  6.7  6.95  7.2  7.45  7.75  8  8.3  8.6  8.95  9.25  9.6  9.95  10.3  10.7  11.05  11.45

FOR EDGE LIFT   0.08 ,   OPTIC DIAMETERS   8 - 8.5 ,   ZONAL CURVATURES ARE
 5.7  5.9  6.1  6.3  6.55  6.75  7  7.25  7.5  7.75  8.05  8.3  8.6  8.9  9.2  9.5  9.85  10.2  10.5

FOR EDGE LIFT   0.08 ,   OPTIC DIAMETERS   8.5 - 9 ,   ZONAL CURVATURES ARE
 5.45  5.6  5.8  6  6.2  6.4  6.65  6.85  7.1  7.3  7.55  7.8  8.05  8.35  8.6  8.9  9.15  9.45  9.8

FOR EDGE LIFT   0.08 ,   OPTIC DIAMETERS   9 - 9.5 ,   ZONAL CURVATURES ARE
 5.25  5.4  5.6  5.75  5.95  6.15  6.35  6.55  6.75  6.95  7.15  7.4  7.65  7.85  8.1  8.35  8.65  8.9  9.2

FOR EDGE LIFT   0.08 ,   OPTIC DIAMETERS   9.5 - 10 ,   ZONAL CURVATURES ARE
 5.15  5.3  5.45  5.6  5.75  5.9  6.1  6.25  6.45  6.65  6.85  7.05  7.3  7.5  7.7  7.95  8.2  8.45  8.7
```

FOR EDGE LIFT 0.09 , OPTIC DIAMETERS 5 - 5.5 , ZONAL CURVATURES ARE

11.2 11.95 12.75 13.6 14.55 15.6 16.7 17.95 19.35 20.9 22.6 24.55 26.8 29.35 32.3 35.75 39.9 44.9 51.1

FOR EDGE LIFT 0.09 , OPTIC DIAMETERS 5.5 - 6 , ZONAL CURVATURES ARE

9.35 9.9 10.45 11.05 11.7 12.4 13.15 13.95 14.8 15.7 16.7 17.8 19 20.3 21.75 23.35 25.1 27.1 29.35

FOR EDGE LIFT 0.09 , OPTIC DIAMETERS 6 - 6.5 , ZONAL CURVATURES ARE

8.15 8.55 9 9.45 9.95 10.45 11 11.6 12.2 12.85 13.55 14.3 15.1 15.95 16.85 17.85 18.9 20.1 21.35

FOR EDGE LIFT 0.09 , OPTIC DIAMETERS 6.5 - 7 , ZONAL CURVATURES ARE

7.3 7.6 8 8.35 8.75 9.15 9.6 10.05 10.55 11.05 11.6 12.15 12.75 13.35 14.05 14.75 15.5 16.3 17.15

FOR EDGE LIFT 0.09 , OPTIC DIAMETERS 7 - 7.5 , ZONAL CURVATURES ARE

6.65 6.95 7.25 7.55 7.9 8.25 8.6 9 9.4 9.8 10.2 10.7 11.15 11.65 12.15 12.7 13.3 13.9 14.55

FOR EDGE LIFT 0.09 , OPTIC DIAMETERS 7.5 - 8 , ZONAL CURVATURES ARE

6.15 6.4 6.7 6.95 7.25 7.55 7.85 8.15 8.5 8.85 9.2 9.6 10 10.4 10.85 11.3 11.75 12.25 12.75

FOR EDGE LIFT 0.09 , OPTIC DIAMETERS 8 - 8.5 , ZONAL CURVATURES ARE

5.8 6 6.25 6.5 6.75 7 7.25 7.55 7.85 8.15 8.45 8.8 9.15 9.5 9.85 10.2 10.6 11.05 11.45

FOR EDGE LIFT 0.09 , OPTIC DIAMETERS 8.5 - 9 , ZONAL CURVATURES ARE

5.5 5.7 5.9 6.1 6.35 6.55 6.8 7.05 7.3 7.6 7.85 8.15 8.45 8.75 9.05 9.4 9.75 10.1 10.45

FOR EDGE LIFT 0.09 , OPTIC DIAMETERS 9 - 9.5 , ZONAL CURVATURES ARE

5.3 5.45 5.65 5.85 6.05 6.25 6.45 6.65 6.9 7.15 7.4 7.65 7.9 8.15 8.45 8.75 9.05 9.35 9.7

FOR EDGE LIFT 0.09 , OPTIC DIAMETERS 9.5 - 10 , ZONAL CURVATURES ARE

5.15 5.3 5.45 5.6 5.8 5.95 6.15 6.35 6.55 6.8 7 7.25 7.45 7.7 7.95 8.2 8.5 8.75 9.05

FOR EDGE LIFT 0.1 , OPTIC DIAMETERS 5 - 5.5 , ZONAL CURVATURES ARE

13.35 14.4 15.65 17 18.5 20.25 22.2 24.5 27.2 30.4 34.25 39 44.95 52.7 63.2 NE NE NE NE

FOR EDGE LIFT 0.1 , OPTIC DIAMETERS 5.5 - 6 , ZONAL CURVATURES ARE

10.55 11.25 12.05 12.85 13.75 14.75 15.85 17.05 18.4 19.9 21.55 23.45 25.6 28.05 30.95 34.3 38.35 43.2 49.25

FOR EDGE LIFT 0.1 , OPTIC DIAMETERS 6 - 6.5 , ZONAL CURVATURES ARE

8.9 9.4 9.95 10.55 11.2 11.85 12.6 13.4 14.25 15.2 16.2 17.3 18.5 19.8 21.3 22.9 24.7 26.75 29.05

FOR EDGE LIFT 0.1 , OPTIC DIAMETERS 6.5 - 7 , ZONAL CURVATURES ARE

7.75 8.15 8.6 9.05 9.55 10.05 10.6 11.2 11.85 12.5 13.2 13.95 14.75 15.65 16.6 17.6 18.7 19.9 21.25

FOR EDGE LIFT 0.1 , OPTIC DIAMETERS 7 - 7.5 , ZONAL CURVATURES ARE

6.95 7.3 7.65 8 8.4 8.85 9.3 9.75 10.25 10.75 11.3 11.85 12.45 13.1 13.8 14.55 15.3 16.15 17.05

FOR EDGE LIFT 0.1 , OPTIC DIAMETERS 7.5 - 8 , ZONAL CURVATURES ARE

6.35 6.65 6.95 7.25 7.6 7.95 8.3 8.7 9.1 9.5 9.95 10.4 10.9 11.4 11.95 12.5 13.1 13.75 14.4

FOR EDGE LIFT 0.1 , OPTIC DIAMETERS 8 - 8.5 , ZONAL CURVATURES ARE

5.9 6.15 6.4 6.7 6.95 7.25 7.55 7.9 8.25 8.6 8.95 9.35 9.75 10.2 10.6 11.1 11.55 12.1 12.6

FOR EDGE LIFT 0.1 , OPTIC DIAMETERS 8.5 - 9 , ZONAL CURVATURES ARE

5.55 5.8 6 6.25 6.5 6.75 7 7.3 7.6 7.9 8.2 8.55 8.9 9.25 9.6 10 10.4 10.85 11.3

FOR EDGE LIFT 0.1 , OPTIC DIAMETERS 9 - 9.5 , ZONAL CURVATURES ARE

5.3 5.5 5.7 5.9 6.1 6.35 6.55 6.8 7.05 7.35 7.6 7.9 8.2 8.5 8.85 9.2 9.55 9.9 10.3

FOR EDGE LIFT 0.1 , OPTIC DIAMETERS 9.5 - 10 , ZONAL CURVATURES ARE

5.15 5.3 5.45 5.65 5.85 6.05 6.25 6.45 6.65 6.9 7.15 7.4 7.65 7.95 8.25 8.55 8.85 9.15 9.5

```
FOR EDGE LIFT   0.11 ,   OPTIC DIAMETERS   5 - 5.5 ,   ZONAL CURVATURES ARE
 16.55  18.3  20.3  22.7  25.55  29  33.3  38.85  46.15  56.3 NE  NE  NE  NE  NE  NE  NE  NE  NE

FOR EDGE LIFT   0.11 ,   OPTIC DIAMETERS   5.5 - 6 ,   ZONAL CURVATURES ARE
 12.2  13.15  14.25  15.45  16.8  18.35  20.1  22.15  24.5  27.25  30.55  34.55  39.45  45.75  54 NE  NE  NE  NE

FOR EDGE LIFT   0.11 ,   OPTIC DIAMETERS   6 - 6.5 ,   ZONAL CURVATURES ARE
 9.8  10.5  11.2  12  12.85  13.8  14.8  15.95  17.2  18.6  20.2  21.95  24  26.3  29  32.15  35.9  40.4  46

FOR EDGE LIFT   0.11 ,   OPTIC DIAMETERS   6.5 - 7 ,   ZONAL CURVATURES ARE
 8.35  8.85  9.35  9.95  10.55  11.2  11.9  12.7  13.5  14.45  15.4  16.5  17.65  18.95  20.4  22  23.8  25.8  28.1

FOR EDGE LIFT   0.11 ,   OPTIC DIAMETERS   7 - 7.5 ,   ZONAL CURVATURES ARE
 7.3  7.7  8.15  8.6  9.05  9.55  10.1  10.65  11.3  11.95  12.65  13.4  14.2  15.1  16.05  17.05  18.15  19.4  20.75

FOR EDGE LIFT   0.11 ,   OPTIC DIAMETERS   7.5 - 8 ,   ZONAL CURVATURES ARE
 6.55  6.9  7.25  7.6  8  8.4  8.85  9.3  9.8  10.3  10.85  11.4  12  12.65  13.35  14.1  14.9  15.75  16.65

FOR EDGE LIFT   0.11 ,   OPTIC DIAMETERS   8 - 8.5 ,   ZONAL CURVATURES ARE
 6.05  6.3  6.6  6.9  7.25  7.55  7.95  8.3  8.7  9.1  9.55  10  10.5  11.05  11.55  12.15  12.75  13.4  14.1

FOR EDGE LIFT   0.11 ,   OPTIC DIAMETERS   8.5 - 9 ,   ZONAL CURVATURES ARE
 5.65  5.85  6.1  6.35  6.65  6.95  7.25  7.55  7.9  8.25  8.6  9  9.4  9.85  10.25  10.75  11.25  11.75  12.3

FOR EDGE LIFT   0.11 ,   OPTIC DIAMETERS   9 - 9.5 ,   ZONAL CURVATURES ARE
 5.35  5.55  5.75  5.95  6.2  6.45  6.7  7  7.25  7.55  7.9  8.2  8.55  8.9  9.3  9.7  10.1  10.55  11

FOR EDGE LIFT   0.11 ,   OPTIC DIAMETERS   9.5 - 10 ,   ZONAL CURVATURES ARE
 5.15  5.3  5.5  5.7  5.9  6.1  6.3  6.55  6.8  7.05  7.35  7.6  7.9  8.2  8.55  8.9  9.25  9.6  10
```

FOR EDGE LIFT 0.12 , OPTIC DIAMETERS 5 - 5.5 , ZONAL CURVATURES ARE

21.9 25.1 29.15 34.4 41.5 51.65 67.3 NE NE NE NE NE NE NE NE NE NE NE NE

FOR EDGE LIFT 0.12 , OPTIC DIAMETERS 5.5 - 6 , ZONAL CURVATURES ARE

14.45 15.9 17.55 19.45 21.75 24.45 27.7 31.75 36.85 43.6 52.75 66.05 NE NE NE NE NE NE NE

FOR EDGE LIFT 0.12 , OPTIC DIAMETERS 6 - 6.5 , ZONAL CURVATURES ARE

11 11.9 12.85 13.95 15.15 16.5 18.05 19.8 21.8 24.15 26.95 30.25 34.3 39.35 45.75 54.25 65.95 NE NE

FOR EDGE LIFT 0.12 , OPTIC DIAMETERS 6.5 - 7 , ZONAL CURVATURES ARE

9 9.65 10.3 11.05 11.85 12.7 13.65 14.7 15.85 17.15 18.6 20.25 22.1 24.2 26.65 29.5 32.85 36.9 41.85

FOR EDGE LIFT 0.12 , OPTIC DIAMETERS 7 - 7.5 , ZONAL CURVATURES ARE

7.7 8.2 8.7 9.25 9.8 10.45 11.15 11.85 12.65 13.5 14.45 15.45 16.6 17.85 19.2 20.75 22.45 24.4 26.6

FOR EDGE LIFT 0.12 , OPTIC DIAMETERS 7.5 - 8 , ZONAL CURVATURES ARE

6.8 7.2 7.6 8.05 8.5 8.95 9.5 10.05 10.65 11.25 11.95 12.7 13.45 14.3 15.25 16.25 17.35 18.55 19.85

FOR EDGE LIFT 0.12 , OPTIC DIAMETERS 8 - 8.5 , ZONAL CURVATURES ARE

6.15 6.5 6.8 7.15 7.55 7.9 8.35 8.8 9.25 9.75 10.25 10.85 11.45 12.1 12.75 13.5 14.3 15.15 16.05

FOR EDGE LIFT 0.12 , OPTIC DIAMETERS 8.5 - 9 , ZONAL CURVATURES ARE

5.7 5.95 6.25 6.5 6.85 7.15 7.5 7.85 8.25 8.65 9.1 9.55 10 10.5 11.05 11.65 12.25 12.9 13.6

FOR EDGE LIFT 0.12 , OPTIC DIAMETERS 9 - 9.5 , ZONAL CURVATURES ARE

5.4 5.6 5.8 6.05 6.3 6.6 6.85 7.15 7.5 7.85 8.2 8.55 8.95 9.4 9.85 10.3 10.8 11.3 11.85

FOR EDGE LIFT 0.12 , OPTIC DIAMETERS 9.5 - 10 , ZONAL CURVATURES ARE

5.15 5.35 5.5 5.7 5.95 6.15 6.4 6.65 6.95 7.2 7.5 7.85 8.15 8.55 8.9 9.3 9.7 10.15 10.6

```
FOR EDGE LIFT   0.13 ,   OPTIC DIAMETERS   5 - 5.5 ,    ZONAL CURVATURES ARE
 32.65  40.4  52.15  71.95 NE  NE  NE  NE  NE  NE  NE  NE  NE  NE  NE  NE  NE  NE  NE

FOR EDGE LIFT   0.13 ,   OPTIC DIAMETERS   5.5 - 6 ,    ZONAL CURVATURES ARE
 17.9  20.2  23  26.45  30.9  36.7  44.75  56.45  75.25 NE  NE  NE  NE  NE  NE  NE  NE  NE  NE

FOR EDGE LIFT   0.13 ,   OPTIC DIAMETERS   6 - 6.5 ,    ZONAL CURVATURES ARE
 12.6  13.8  15.15  16.75  18.55  20.7  23.2  26.25  30  34.7  40.85  49.1  60.8  78.8 NE  NE  NE  NE  NE

FOR EDGE LIFT   0.13 ,   OPTIC DIAMETERS   6.5 - 7 ,    ZONAL CURVATURES ARE
 9.9  10.65  11.5  12.45  13.55  14.7  16.05  17.55  19.3  21.3  23.6  26.35  29.6  33.6  38.6  45  53.4  65.15  82.5

FOR EDGE LIFT   0.13 ,   OPTIC DIAMETERS   7 - 7.5 ,    ZONAL CURVATURES ARE
 8.2  8.8  9.4  10.05  10.8  11.55  12.45  13.4  14.45  15.6  16.95  18.4  20.05  21.95  24.1  26.6  29.55  33.05  37.3

FOR EDGE LIFT   0.13 ,   OPTIC DIAMETERS   7.5 - 8 ,    ZONAL CURVATURES ARE
 7.1  7.55  8  8.5  9.05  9.65  10.25  10.95  11.7  12.5  13.35  14.3  15.35  16.55  17.8  19.25  20.85  22.65  24.7

FOR EDGE LIFT   0.13 ,   OPTIC DIAMETERS   8 - 8.5 ,    ZONAL CURVATURES ARE
 6.35  6.7  7.05  7.45  7.85  8.35  8.8  9.35  9.9  10.5  11.15  11.85  12.6  13.4  14.3  15.25  16.3  17.45  18.7

FOR EDGE LIFT   0.13 ,   OPTIC DIAMETERS   8.5 - 9 ,    ZONAL CURVATURES ARE
 5.8  6.05  6.35  6.7  7.05  7.4  7.8  8.2  8.65  9.1  9.65  10.15  10.75  11.35  12  12.75  13.5  14.3  15.2

FOR EDGE LIFT   0.13 ,   OPTIC DIAMETERS   9 - 9.5 ,    ZONAL CURVATURES ARE
 5.4  5.65  5.9  6.15  6.4  6.7  7.05  7.4  7.75  8.15  8.55  9  9.45  9.95  10.45  11  11.6  12.25  12.9

FOR EDGE LIFT   0.13 ,   OPTIC DIAMETERS   9.5 - 10 ,    ZONAL CURVATURES ARE
 5.15  5.35  5.55  5.75  6  6.25  6.5  6.8  7.1  7.4  7.75  8.1  8.5  8.9  9.3  9.75  10.25  10.75  11.3
```

```
FOR EDGE LIFT   0.14 ,   OPTIC DIAMETERS   5  -  5.5 ,    ZONAL CURVATURES ARE
NE  NE  NE  NE  NE  NE  NE  NE  NE  NE  NE  NE  NE  NE  NE  NE  NE  NE  NE

FOR EDGE LIFT   0.14 ,   OPTIC DIAMETERS   5.5  -  6 ,    ZONAL CURVATURES ARE
 23.55  27.8  33.55  41.6  53.85 NE  NE  NE  NE  NE  NE  NE  NE  NE  NE  NE  NE  NE  NE

FOR EDGE LIFT   0.14 ,   OPTIC DIAMETERS   6  -  6.5 ,    ZONAL CURVATURES ARE
 14.8  16.55  18.6  21.05  24.1  27.85  32.75  39.25  48.4  62.1 NE  NE  NE  NE  NE  NE  NE  NE  NE

FOR EDGE LIFT   0.14 ,   OPTIC DIAMETERS   6.5  -  7 ,    ZONAL CURVATURES ARE
 10.95  11.95  13.1  14.4  15.85  17.55  19.55  21.9  24.75  28.2  32.45  38  45.3  55.55 NE  NE  NE  NE  NE

FOR EDGE LIFT   0.14 ,   OPTIC DIAMETERS   7  -  7.5 ,    ZONAL CURVATURES ARE
 8.8  9.5  10.25  11.05  12  13  14.15  15.45  16.95  18.6  20.55  22.8  25.45  28.65  32.55  37.35  43.55  51.7  63

FOR EDGE LIFT   0.14 ,   OPTIC DIAMETERS   7.5  -  8 ,    ZONAL CURVATURES ARE
 7.45  7.95  8.5  9.1  9.75  10.45  11.25  12.1  13.05  14.05  15.25  16.55  18  19.65  21.55  23.7  26.25  29.25  32.8

FOR EDGE LIFT   0.14 ,   OPTIC DIAMETERS   8  -  8.5 ,    ZONAL CURVATURES ARE
 6.5  6.9  7.3  7.8  8.25  8.8  9.4  10  10.7  11.4  12.2  13.1  14.05  15.15  16.3  17.6  19.05  20.7  22.55

FOR EDGE LIFT   0.14 ,   OPTIC DIAMETERS   8.5  -  9 ,    ZONAL CURVATURES ARE
 5.9  6.2  6.5  6.9  7.25  7.7  8.15  8.6  9.1  9.7  10.3  10.95  11.65  12.4  13.2  14.1  15.1  16.2  17.35

FOR EDGE LIFT   0.14 ,   OPTIC DIAMETERS   9  -  9.5 ,    ZONAL CURVATURES ARE
 5.45  5.7  5.95  6.25  6.55  6.9  7.25  7.6  8.05  8.45  8.95  9.45  10  10.6  11.2  11.85 '12.6  13.4  14.25

FOR EDGE LIFT   0.14 ,   OPTIC DIAMETERS   9.5  -  10 ,    ZONAL CURVATURES ARE
 5.2  5.35  5.55  5.8  6.05  6.3  6.6  6.9  7.25  7.6  8  8.4  8.8  9.3  9.8  10.3  10.9  11.5  12.15
```

FOR EDGE LIFT 0.15 , OPTIC DIAMETERS 5 - 5.5 , ZONAL CURVATURES ARE

NE NE NE NE NE NE NE NE NE NE NE NE NE NE NE NE NE NE NE

FOR EDGE LIFT 0.15 , OPTIC DIAMETERS 5.5 - 6 , ZONAL CURVATURES ARE

34.8 45.05 62.45 NE NE NE NE NE NE NE NE NE NE NE NE NE NE NE NE

FOR EDGE LIFT 0.15 , OPTIC DIAMETERS 6 - 6.5 , ZONAL CURVATURES ARE

18.05 20.75 24.15 28.55 34.55 43 56 NE NE NE NE NE NE NE NE NE NE NE NE

FOR EDGE LIFT 0.15 , OPTIC DIAMETERS 6.5 - 7 , ZONAL CURVATURES ARE

12.35 13.7 15.3 17.1 19.3 21.95 25.2 29.3 34.7 42 52.45 NE NE NE NE NE NE NE NE

FOR EDGE LIFT 0.15 , OPTIC DIAMETERS 7 - 7.5 , ZONAL CURVATURES ARE

9.5 10.35 11.3 12.35 13.6 14.95 16.55 18.4 20.55 23.15 26.3 30.15 35.1 41.55 50.4 63.15 NE NE NE

FOR EDGE LIFT 0.15 , OPTIC DIAMETERS 7.5 - 8 , ZONAL CURVATURES ARE

7.8 8.4 9.05 9.8 10.6 11.45 12.45 13.55 14.8 16.2 17.8 19.65 21.8 24.35 27.4 31.1 35.7 41.55 49.2

FOR EDGE LIFT 0.15 , OPTIC DIAMETERS 8 - 8.5 , ZONAL CURVATURES ARE

6.7 7.15 7.65 8.15 8.75 9.35 10.05 10.8 11.65 12.55 13.6 14.75 16 17.45 19.05 20.95 23.1 25.6 28.55

FOR EDGE LIFT 0.15 , OPTIC DIAMETERS 8.5 - 9 , ZONAL CURVATURES ARE

5.95 6.3 6.7 7.1 7.5 8 8.5 9.05 9.7 10.35 11.05 11.85 12.75 13.7 14.75 15.9 17.2 18.7 20.35

FOR EDGE LIFT 0.15 , OPTIC DIAMETERS 9 - 9.5 , ZONAL CURVATURES ARE

5.5 5.75 6.05 6.35 6.7 7.05 7.45 7.9 8.35 8.85 9.4 10 10.65 11.35 12.1 12.95 13.85 14.85 15.9

FOR EDGE LIFT 0.15 , OPTIC DIAMETERS 9.5 - 10 , ZONAL CURVATURES ARE

5.2 5.4 5.6 5.85 6.1 6.4 6.7 7.05 7.45 7.85 8.25 8.7 9.2 9.75 10.35 10.95 11.65 12.35 13.15

TABLE II Back Peripheral Optic Radii (Zonal Curvatures) for the following:
BCOR 5.1 to 6.9 in 0.1 steps
Zone Width 0.5 Zone Inner Diameters 5.0 to 9.5 in 0.5 steps
Axial Edge Lift Components 0.01 to 0.15 in 0.01 steps

FOR EDGE LIFT 0.01 , OPTIC DIAMETERS 5 - 6 , ZONAL CURVATURES ARE

5.2 5.3 5.45 5.55 5.65 5.75 5.85 5.95 6.1 6.2 6.3 6.4 6.5 6.65 6.75 6.85 6.95 7.05 7.2

FOR EDGE LIFT 0.01 , OPTIC DIAMETERS 5.5 - 6.5 , ZONAL CURVATURES ARE

5.2 5.3 5.4 5.5 5.6 5.75 5.85 5.95 6.05 6.15 6.25 6.4 6.5 6.6 6.7 6.8 6.9 7.05 7.15

FOR EDGE LIFT 0.01 , OPTIC DIAMETERS 6 - 7 , ZONAL CURVATURES ARE

5.15 5.3 5.4 5.5 5.6 5.7 5.8 5.9 6.05 6.15 6.25 6.35 6.45 6.55 6.65 6.8 6.9 7 7.1

FOR EDGE LIFT 0.01 , OPTIC DIAMETERS 6.5 - 7.5 , ZONAL CURVATURES ARE

5.15 5.25 5.35 5.45 5.6 5.7 5.8 5.9 6 6.1 6.2 6.35 6.45 6.55 6.65 6.75 6.85 6.95 7.1

FOR EDGE LIFT 0.01 , OPTIC DIAMETERS 7 - 8 , ZONAL CURVATURES ARE

5.15 5.25 5.35 5.45 5.55 5.65 5.8 5.9 6 6.1 6.2 6.3 6.4 6.5 6.65 6.75 6.85 6.95 7.05

FOR EDGE LIFT 0.01 , OPTIC DIAMETERS 7.5 - 8.5 , ZONAL CURVATURES ARE

5.15 5.25 5.35 5.45 5.55 5.65 5.75 5.85 5.95 6.1 6.2 6.3 6.4 6.5 6.6 6.7 6.8 6.95 7.05

FOR EDGE LIFT 0.01 , OPTIC DIAMETERS 8 - 9 , ZONAL CURVATURES ARE

5.1 5.2 5.35 5.45 5.55 5.65 5.75 5.85 5.95 6.05 6.15 6.25 6.4 6.5 6.6 6.7 6.8 6.9 7

FOR EDGE LIFT 0.01 , OPTIC DIAMETERS 8.5 - 9.5 , ZONAL CURVATURES ARE

5.1 5.2 5.3 5.4 5.5 5.65 5.75 5.85 5.95 6.05 6.15 6.25 6.35 6.45 6.55 6.7 6.8 6.9 7

FOR EDGE LIFT 0.01 , OPTIC DIAMETERS 9 - 10 , ZONAL CURVATURES ARE

5.1 5.2 5.3 5.4 5.5 5.6 5.7 5.85 5.95 6.05 6.15 6.25 6.35 6.45 6.55 6.65 6.75 6.85 7

FOR EDGE LIFT 0.01 , OPTIC DIAMETERS 9.5 - 10.5 , ZONAL CURVATURES ARE

NE NE 5.3 5.4 5.5 5.6 5.7 5.8 5.9 6 6.15 6.25 6.35 6.45 6.55 6.65 6.75 6.85 6.95

```
FOR EDGE LIFT   0.02 ,   OPTIC DIAMETERS   5 - 6 ,   ZONAL CURVATURES ARE
5.35  5.45  5.55  5.7  5.8  5.95  6.05  6.15  6.3  6.4  6.5  6.65  6.75  6.9  7  7.1  7.25  7.35  7.5

FOR EDGE LIFT   0.02 ,   OPTIC DIAMETERS   5.5 - 6.5 ,   ZONAL CURVATURES ARE
5.3  5.4  5.5  5.65  5.75  5.85  6  6.1  6.2  6.35  6.45  6.55  6.7  6.8  6.95  7.05  7.15  7.3  7.4

FOR EDGE LIFT   0.02 ,   OPTIC DIAMETERS   6 - 7 ,   ZONAL CURVATURES ARE
5.25  5.35  5.5  5.6  5.7  5.8  5.95  6.05  6.15  6.3  6.4  6.5  6.65  6.75  6.85  7  7.1  7.2  7.35

FOR EDGE LIFT   0.02 ,   OPTIC DIAMETERS   6.5 - 7.5 ,   ZONAL CURVATURES ARE
5.2  5.35  5.45  5.55  5.65  5.8  5.9  6  6.1  6.25  6.35  6.45  6.6  6.7  6.8  6.95  7.05  7.15  7.3

FOR EDGE LIFT   0.02 ,   OPTIC DIAMETERS   7 - 8 ,   ZONAL CURVATURES ARE
5.2  5.3  5.4  5.5  5.65  5.75  5.85  5.95  6.1  6.2  6.3  6.4  6.55  6.65  6.75  6.9  7  7.1  7.2

FOR EDGE LIFT   0.02 ,   OPTIC DIAMETERS   7.5 - 8.5 ,   ZONAL CURVATURES ARE
5.15  5.25  5.4  5.5  5.6  5.7  5.8  5.95  6.05  6.15  6.25  6.4  6.5  6.6  6.7  6.85  6.95  7.05  7.15

FOR EDGE LIFT   0.02 ,   OPTIC DIAMETERS   8 - 9 ,   ZONAL CURVATURES ARE
5.15  5.25  5.35  5.45  5.55  5.7  5.8  5.9  6  6.1  6.25  6.35  6.45  6.55  6.7  6.8  6.9  7  7.15

FOR EDGE LIFT   0.02 ,   OPTIC DIAMETERS   8.5 - 9.5 ,   ZONAL CURVATURES ARE
5.1  5.25  5.35  5.45  5.55  5.65  5.75  5.9  6  6.1  6.2  6.3  6.45  6.55  6.65  6.75  6.85  7  7.1

FOR EDGE LIFT   0.02 ,   OPTIC DIAMETERS   9 - 10 ,   ZONAL CURVATURES ARE
5.1  5.2  5.3  5.4  5.55  5.65  5.75  5.85  5.95  6.05  6.2  6.3  6.4  6.5  6.6  6.75  6.85  6.95  7.05

FOR EDGE LIFT   0.02 ,   OPTIC DIAMETERS   9.5 - 10.5 ,   ZONAL CURVATURES ARE
NE  NE  5.3  5.4  5.5  5.6  5.75  5.85  5.95  6.05  6.15  6.25  6.35  6.5  6.6  6.7  6.8  6.9  7.05
```

```
FOR EDGE LIFT    0.03 ,    OPTIC DIAMETERS    5  -  6 ,     ZONAL CURVATURES ARE

 5.5  5.6  5.75  5.85  6  6.1  6.25  6.35  6.5  6.65  6.75  6.9  7.05  7.15  7.3  7.45  7.55  7.7  7.85

FOR EDGE LIFT    0.03 ,    OPTIC DIAMETERS    5.5  -  6.5 ,     ZONAL CURVATURES ARE

 5.4  5.5  5.65  5.75  5.9  6  6.15  6.25  6.4  6.55  6.65  6.8  6.9  7.05  7.15  7.3  7.45  7.55  7.7

FOR EDGE LIFT    0.03 ,    OPTIC DIAMETERS    6  -  7 ,     ZONAL CURVATURES ARE

 5.35  5.45  5.6  5.7  5.8  5.95  6.05  6.2  6.3  6.45  6.55  6.7  6.8  6.95  7.05  7.2  7.35  7.45  7.6

FOR EDGE LIFT    0.03 ,    OPTIC DIAMETERS    6.5  -  7.5 ,     ZONAL CURVATURES ARE

 5.3  5.4  5.5  5.65  5.75  5.9  6  6.1  6.25  6.35  6.5  6.6  6.75  6.85  7  7.1  7.25  7.35  7.5

FOR EDGE LIFT    0.03 ,    OPTIC DIAMETERS    7  -  8 ,     ZONAL CURVATURES ARE

 5.25  5.35  5.45  5.6  5.7  5.8  5.95  6.05  6.2  6.3  6.4  6.55  6.65  6.8  6.9  7.05  7.15  7.3  7.4

FOR EDGE LIFT    0.03 ,    OPTIC DIAMETERS    7.5  -  8.5 ,     ZONAL CURVATURES ARE

 5.2  5.3  5.4  5.55  5.65  5.75  5.9  6  6.1  6.25  6.35  6.5  6.6  6.7  6.85  6.95  7.1  7.2  7.35

FOR EDGE LIFT    0.03 ,    OPTIC DIAMETERS    8  -  9 ,     ZONAL CURVATURES ARE

 5.15  5.25  5.4  5.5  5.6  5.75  5.85  5.95  6.05  6.2  6.3  6.4  6.55  6.65  6.8  6.9  7  7.15  7.25

FOR EDGE LIFT    0.03 ,    OPTIC DIAMETERS    8.5  -  9.5 ,     ZONAL CURVATURES ARE

 5.15  5.25  5.35  5.45  5.6  5.7  5.8  5.9  6.05  6.15  6.25  6.4  6.5  6.6  6.75  6.85  6.95  7.1  7.2

FOR EDGE LIFT    0.03 ,    OPTIC DIAMETERS    9  -  10 ,     ZONAL CURVATURES ARE

 5.1  5.2  5.35  5.45  5.55  5.65  5.75  5.9  6  6.1  6.2  6.35  6.45  6.55  6.7  6.8  6.9  7.05  7.15

FOR EDGE LIFT    0.03 ,    OPTIC DIAMETERS    9.5  -  10.5 ,     ZONAL CURVATURES ARE

NE  NE   5.3  5.4  5.5  5.65  5.75  5.85  5.95  6.05  6.2  6.3  6.4  6.5  6.65  6.75  6.85  7  7.1
```

```
FOR EDGE LIFT   0.04 ,   OPTIC DIAMETERS   5  -  6 ,    ZONAL CURVATURES ARE
 5.6  5.75  5.9  6.05  6.15  6.3  6.45  6.6  6.75  6.9  7.05  7.15  7.3  7.45  7.6  7.75  7.9  8.05  8.25

FOR EDGE LIFT   0.04 ,   OPTIC DIAMETERS   5.5  -  6.5 ,    ZONAL CURVATURES ARE
 5.5  5.65  5.8  5.9  6.05  6.2  6.3  6.45  6.6  6.75  6.85  7  7.15  7.3  7.45  7.6  7.75  7.9  8.05

FOR EDGE LIFT   0.04 ,   OPTIC DIAMETERS   6  -  7 ,    ZONAL CURVATURES ARE
 5.45  5.55  5.7  5.8  5.95  6.05  6.2  6.35  6.45  6.6  6.75  6.9  7  7.15  7.3  7.45  7.6  7.7  7.85

FOR EDGE LIFT   0.04 ,   OPTIC DIAMETERS   6.5  -  7.5 ,    ZONAL CURVATURES ARE
 5.35  5.5  5.6  5.75  5.85  6  6.1  6.25  6.35  6.5  6.65  6.75  6.9  7.05  7.15  7.3  7.45  7.6  7.7

FOR EDGE LIFT   0.04 ,   OPTIC DIAMETERS   7  -  8 ,    ZONAL CURVATURES ARE
 5.3  5.4  5.55  5.65  5.8  5.9  6.05  6.15  6.3  6.4  6.55  6.65  6.8  6.95  7.05  7.2  7.35  7.45  7.6

FOR EDGE LIFT   0.04 ,   OPTIC DIAMETERS   7.5  -  8.5 ,    ZONAL CURVATURES ARE
 5.25  5.35  5.45  5.6  5.7  5.85  5.95  6.1  6.2  6.35  6.45  6.6  6.7  6.85  6.95  7.1  7.25  7.35  7.5

FOR EDGE LIFT   0.04 ,   OPTIC DIAMETERS   8  -  9 ,    ZONAL CURVATURES ARE
 5.2  5.3  5.4  5.55  5.65  5.75  5.9  6  6.15  6.25  6.4  6.5  6.65  6.75  6.9  7  7.15  7.25  7.4

FOR EDGE LIFT   0.04 ,   OPTIC DIAMETERS   8.5  -  9.5 ,    ZONAL CURVATURES ARE
 5.15  5.25  5.35  5.5  5.6  5.7  5.85  5.95  6.1  6.2  6.3  6.45  6.55  6.7  6.8  6.95  7.05  7.2  7.3

FOR EDGE LIFT   0.04 ,   OPTIC DIAMETERS   9  -  10 ,    ZONAL CURVATURES ARE
 5.1  5.25  5.35  5.45  5.55  5.7  5.8  5.9  6.05  6.15  6.25  6.4  6.5  6.65  6.75  6.85  7  7.1  7.25

FOR EDGE LIFT   0.04 ,   OPTIC DIAMETERS   9.5  -  10.5 ,    ZONAL CURVATURES ARE
NE  NE   5.3  5.4  5.55  5.65  5.75  5.85  6  6.1  6.2  6.35  6.45  6.55  6.7  6.8  6.95  7.05  7.15
```

FOR EDGE LIFT 0.05 , OPTIC DIAMETERS 5 - 6 , ZONAL CURVATURES ARE

5.8 5.95 6.1 6.25 6.4 6.55 6.7 6.85 7 7.15 7.3 7.5 7.65 7.8 8 8.15 8.3 8.5 8.65

FOR EDGE LIFT 0.05 , OPTIC DIAMETERS 5.5 - 6.5 , ZONAL CURVATURES ARE

5.65 5.8 5.9 6.05 6.2 6.35 6.5 6.65 6.8 6.95 7.1 7.25 7.4 7.6 7.75 7.9 8.05 8.2 8.4

FOR EDGE LIFT 0.05 , OPTIC DIAMETERS 6 - 7 , ZONAL CURVATURES ARE

5.5 5.65 5.8 5.95 6.1 6.2 6.35 6.5 6.65 6.8 6.95 7.1 7.25 7.4 7.55 7.7 7.85 8 8.15

FOR EDGE LIFT 0.05 , OPTIC DIAMETERS 6.5 - 7.5 , ZONAL CURVATURES ARE

5.4 5.55 5.7 5.8 5.95 6.1 6.25 6.35 6.5 6.65 6.8 6.95 7.1 7.25 7.35 7.5 7.65 7.8 7.95

FOR EDGE LIFT 0.05 , OFTIC DIAMETERS 7 - 8 , ZONAL CURVATURES ARE

5.35 5.45 5.6 5.75 5.85 6 6.1 6.25 6.4 6.55 6.65 6.8 6.95 7.1 7.25 7.35 7.5 7.65 7.8

FOR EDGE LIFT 0.05 , OFTIC DIAMETERS 7.5 - 8.5 , ZONAL CURVATURES ARE

5.25 5.4 5.5 5.65 5.75 5.9 6.05 6.15 6.3 6.45 6.55 6.7 6.85 6.95 7.1 7.25 7.4 7.5 7.65

FOR EDGE LIFT 0.05 , OPTIC DIAMETERS 8 - 9 , ZONAL CURVATURES ARE

5.2 5.35 5.45 5.55 5.7 5.8 5.95 6.1 6.2 6.35 6.45 6.6 6.75 6.85 7 7.15 7.25 7.4 7.55

FOR EDGE LIFT 0.05 , OPTIC DIAMETERS 8.5 - 9.5 , ZONAL CURVATURES ARE

5.15 5.3 5.4 5.5 5.65 5.75 5.9 6 6.15 6.25 6.4 6.5 6.65 6.75 6.9 7.05 7.15 7.3 7.45

FOR EDGE LIFT 0.05 , OPTIC DIAMETERS 9 - 10 , ZONAL CURVATURES ARE

5.1 5.25 5.35 5.45 5.6 5.7 5.8 5.95 6.05 6.2 6.3 6.45 6.55 6.7 6.8 6.95 7.05 7.2 7.35

FOR EDGE LIFT 0.05 , OPTIC DIAMETERS 9.5 - 10.5 , ZONAL CURVATURES ARE

NE NE 5.3 5.4 5.55 5.65 5.75 5.9 6 6.15 6.25 6.35 6.5 6.6 6.75 6.85 7 7.1 7.25

```
FOR EDGE LIFT   6.00000E-2 ,   OPTIC DIAMETERS   5  -  6 ,    ZONAL CURVATURES ARE
 5.95  6.1  6.25  6.45  6.6  6.75  6.95  7.1  7.3  7.45  7.65  7.85  8  8.2  8.4  8.55  8.75  8.95  9.15

FOR EDGE LIFT   6.00000E-2 ,   OPTIC DIAMETERS   5.5  -  6.5 ,    ZONAL CURVATURES ARE
 5.75  5.9  6.1  6.25  6.4  6.55  6.7  6.9  7.05  7.2  7.35  7.55  7.7  7.9  8.05  8.25  8.4  8.6  8.8

FOR EDGE LIFT   6.00000E-2 ,   OPTIC DIAMETERS   6  -  7 ,    ZONAL CURVATURES ARE
 5.6  5.75  5.9  6.05  6.2  6.35  6.5  6.7  6.85  7  7.15  7.3  7.5  7.65  7.8  8  8.15  8.3  8.5

FOR EDGE LIFT   6.00000E-2 ,   OPTIC DIAMETERS   6.5  -  7.5 ,    ZONAL CURVATURES ARE
 5.5  5.65  5.8  5.9  6.05  6.2  6.35  6.5  6.65  6.8  6.95  7.1  7.3  7.45  7.6  7.75  7.9  8.1  8.25

FOR EDGE LIFT   6.00000E-2 ,   OPTIC DIAMETERS   7  -  8 ,    ZONAL CURVATURES ARE
 5.4  5.55  5.65  5.8  5.95  6.1  6.25  6.35  6.5  6.65  6.8  6.95  7.1  7.25  7.4  7.55  7.7  7.85  8.05

FOR EDGE LIFT   6.00000E-2 ,   OPTIC DIAMETERS   7.5  -  8.5 ,    ZONAL CURVATURES ARE
 5.3  5.45  5.55  5.7  5.85  5.95  6.1  6.25  6.4  6.55  6.65  6.8  6.95  7.1  7.25  7.4  7.55  7.7  7.85

FOR EDGE LIFT   6.00000E-2 ,   OPTIC DIAMETERS   8  -  9 ,    ZONAL CURVATURES ARE
 5.25  5.35  5.5  5.6  5.75  5.85  6  6.15  6.3  6.4  6.55  6.7  6.85  6.95  7.1  7.25  7.4  7.55  7.7

FOR EDGE LIFT   6.00000E-2 ,   OPTIC DIAMETERS   8.5  -  9.5 ,    ZONAL CURVATURES ARE
 5.15  5.3  5.4  5.55  5.65  5.8  5.9  6.05  6.2  6.3  6.45  6.6  6.7  6.85  7  7.15  7.25  7.4  7.55

FOR EDGE LIFT   6.00000E-2 ,   OPTIC DIAMETERS   9  -  10 ,    ZONAL CURVATURES ARE
 5.1  5.25  5.35  5.5  5.6  5.7  5.85  5.95  6.1  6.25  6.35  6.5  6.6  6.75  6.9  7  7.15  7.3  7.45

FOR EDGE LIFT   6.00000E-2 ,   OPTIC DIAMETERS   9.5  -  10.5 ,    ZONAL CURVATURES ARE
NE  NE   5.3  5.45  5.55  5.65  5.8  5.9  6.05  6.15  6.3  6.4  6.55  6.65  6.8  6.95  7.05  7.2  7.35
```

```
FOR EDGE LIFT   0.07 ,   OPTIC DIAMETERS   5 - 6 ,   ZONAL CURVATURES ARE
 6.15  6.3  6.5  6.65  6.85  7.05  7.25  7.4  7.6  7.8  8  8.2  8.4  8.65  8.85  9.05  9.3  9.5  9.7

FOR EDGE LIFT   0.07 ,   OPTIC DIAMETERS   5.5 - 6.5 ,   ZONAL CURVATURES ARE
 5.9  6.1  6.25  6.4  6.6  6.75  6.95  7.1  7.3  7.5  7.65  7.85  8.05  8.25  8.45  8.65  8.85  9.05  9.25

FOR EDGE LIFT   0.07 ,   OPTIC DIAMETERS   6 - 7 ,   ZONAL CURVATURES ARE
 5.75  5.9  6.05  6.2  6.35  6.55  6.7  6.85  7.05  7.2  7.4  7.55  7.75  7.9  8.1  8.3  8.5  8.65  8.85

FOR EDGE LIFT   0.07 ,   OPTIC DIAMETERS   6.5 - 7.5 ,   ZONAL CURVATURES ARE
 5.6  5.75  5.9  6.05  6.2  6.35  6.5  6.65  6.8  7  7.15  7.3  7.5  7.65  7.85  8  8.2  8.35  8.55

FOR EDGE LIFT   0.07 ,   OPTIC DIAMETERS   7 - 8 ,   ZONAL CURVATURES ARE
 5.45  5.6  5.75  5.9  6.05  6.2  6.35  6.5  6.65  6.8  6.95  7.1  7.3  7.45  7.6  7.75  7.95  8.1  8.3

FOR EDGE LIFT   0.07 ,   OPTIC DIAMETERS   7.5 - 8.5 ,   ZONAL CURVATURES ARE
 5.35  5.5  5.6  5.75  5.9  6.05  6.2  6.35  6.5  6.65  6.8  6.95  7.1  7.25  7.4  7.55  7.75  7.9  8.05

FOR EDGE LIFT   0.07 ,   OPTIC DIAMETERS   8 - 9 ,   ZONAL CURVATURES ARE
 5.25  5.4  5.5  5.65  5.8  5.95  6.05  6.2  6.35  6.5  6.65  6.8  6.95  7.1  7.25  7.4  7.55  7.7  7.85

FOR EDGE LIFT   0.07 ,   OPTIC DIAMETERS   8.5 - 9.5 ,   ZONAL CURVATURES ARE
 5.2  5.3  5.45  5.55  5.7  5.85  5.95  6.1  6.25  6.4  6.5  6.65  6.8  6.95  7.1  7.25  7.4  7.55  7.7

FOR EDGE LIFT   0.07 ,   OPTIC DIAMETERS   9 - 10 ,   ZONAL CURVATURES ARE
 5.15  5.25  5.35  5.5  5.6  5.75  5.9  6  6.15  6.25  6.4  6.55  6.7  6.85  6.95  7.1  7.25  7.4  7.55

FOR EDGE LIFT   0.07 ,   OPTIC DIAMETERS   9.5 - 10.5 ,   ZONAL CURVATURES ARE
NE  NE  5.3  5.45  5.55  5.7  5.8  5.95  6.05  6.2  6.3  6.45  6.6  6.7  6.85  7  7.15  7.25  7.4
```

```
FOR EDGE LIFT   0.08 ,   OPTIC DIAMETERS   5  -  6 ,   ZONAL CURVATURES ARE
 6.35  6.55  6.75  6.95  7.15  7.35  7.55  7.75  7.95  8.2  8.4  8.65  8.9  9.1  9.35  9.6  9.85  10.1  10.4

FOR EDGE LIFT   0.08 ,   OPTIC DIAMETERS   5.5  -  6.5 ,   ZONAL CURVATURES ARE
 6.05  6.25  6.45  6.6  6.8  7  7.2  7.4  7.6  7.8  8  8.2  8.4  8.6  8.85  9.05  9.3  9.5  9.75

FOR EDGE LIFT   0.08 ,   OPTIC DIAMETERS   6  -  7 ,   ZONAL CURVATURES ARE
 5.85  6  6.2  6.35  6.55  6.7  6.9  7.05  7.25  7.45  7.65  7.85  8.05  8.25  8.45  8.65  8.85  9.05  9.25

FOR EDGE LIFT   0.08 ,   OPTIC DIAMETERS   6.5  -  7.5 ,   ZONAL CURVATURES ARE
 5.65  5.8  6  6.15  6.3  6.5  6.65  6.8  7  7.15  7.35  7.55  7.7  7.9  8.1  8.3  8.5  8.7  8.9

FOR EDGE LIFT   0.08 ,   OPTIC DIAMETERS   7  -  8 ,   ZONAL CURVATURES ARE
 5.5  5.65  5.8  5.95  6.15  6.3  6.45  6.6  6.8  6.95  7.1  7.3  7.45  7.65  7.8  8  8.2  8.35  8.55

FOR EDGE LIFT   0.08 ,   OPTIC DIAMETERS   7.5  -  8.5 ,   ZONAL CURVATURES ARE
 5.4  5.55  5.7  5.8  5.95  6.1  6.3  6.45  6.6  6.75  6.9  7.05  7.25  7.4  7.6  7.75  7.9  8.1  8.3

FOR EDGE LIFT   0.08 ,   OPTIC DIAMETERS   8  -  9 ,   ZONAL CURVATURES ARE
 5.3  5.4  5.55  5.7  5.85  6  6.15  6.3  6.45  6.6  6.75  6.9  7.05  7.2  7.35  7.55  7.7  7.85  8.05

FOR EDGE LIFT   0.08 ,   OPTIC DIAMETERS   8.5  -  9.5 ,   ZONAL CURVATURES ARE
 5.2  5.35  5.45  5.6  5.75  5.85  6  6.15  6.3  6.45  6.6  6.75  6.9  7.05  7.2  7.35  7.5  7.7  7.85

FOR EDGE LIFT   0.08 ,   OPTIC DIAMETERS   9  -  10 ,   ZONAL CURVATURES ARE
 5.15  5.25  5.4  5.5  5.65  5.75  5.9  6.05  6.2  6.3  6.45  6.6  6.75  6.9  7.05  7.2  7.35  7.5  7.65

FOR EDGE LIFT   0.08 ,   OPTIC DIAMETERS   9.5  -  10.5 ,   ZONAL CURVATURES ARE
NE  NE  5.3  5.45  5.55  5.7  5.8  5.95  6.1  6.2  6.35  6.5  6.65  6.75  6.9  7.05  7.2  7.35  7.5
```

FOR EDGE LIFT 0.09 , OPTIC DIAMETERS 5 - 6 , ZONAL CURVATURES ARE

6.55 6.8 7 7.2 7.45 7.65 7.9 8.15 8.4 8.65 8.9 9.15 9.4 9.7 9.95 10.25 10.55 10.85 11.15

FOR EDGE LIFT 0.09 , OPTIC DIAMETERS 5.5 - 6.5 , ZONAL CURVATURES ARE

6.25 6.45 6.65 6.85 7.05 7.25 7.45 7.65 7.9 8.1 8.35 8.55 8.8 9.05 9.3 9.55 9.8 10.05 10.35

FOR EDGE LIFT 0.09 , CPTIC DIAMETERS 6 - 7 , ZONAL CURVATURES ARE

5.95 6.15 6.35 6.5 6.7 6.9 7.1 7.3 7.5 7.7 7.9 8.15 8.35 8.55 8.8 9 9.25 9.5 9.75

FOR EDGE LIFT 0.09 , OPTIC DIAMETERS 6.5 - 7.5 , ZONAL CURVATURES ARE

5.75 5.95 6.1 6.25 6.45 6.65 6.8 7 7.2 7.4 7.55 7.75 7.95 8.15 8.4 8.6 8.8 9 9.25

FOR EDGE LIFT 0.09 , OPTIC DIAMETERS 7 - 8 , ZONAL CURVATURES ARE

5.6 5.75 5.9 6.05 6.25 6.4 6.55 6.75 6.9 7.1 7.3 7.45 7.65 7.85 8.05 8.25 8.45 8.65 8.85

FOR EDGE LIFT 0.09 , OPTIC DIAMETERS 7.5 - 8.5 , ZONAL CURVATURES ARE

5.45 5.6 5.75 5.9 6.05 6.2 6.35 6.55 6.7 6.85 7.05 7.2 7.4 7.6 7.75 7.95 8.15 8.3 8.5

FOR EDGE LIFT 0.09 , OPTIC DIAMETERS 8 - 9 , ZONAL CURVATURES ARE

5.3 5.45 5.6 5.75 5.9 6.05 6.2 6.35 6.5 6.7 6.85 7 7.15 7.35 7.5 7.7 7.85 8.05 8.25

FOR EDGE LIFT 0.09 , OPTIC DIAMETERS 8.5 - 9.5 , ZONAL CURVATURES ARE

5.2 5.35 5.5 5.6 5.75 5.9 6.05 6.2 6.35 6.5 6.65 6.8 7 7.15 7.3 7.5 7.65 7.8 8

FOR EDGE LIFT 0.09 , OPTIC DIAMETERS 9 - 10 , ZONAL CURVATURES ARE

5.15 5.25 5.4 5.5 5.65 5.8 5.95 6.1 6.2 6.35 6.5 6.65 6.8 7 7.15 7.3 7.45 7.6 7.8

FOR EDGE LIFT 0.09 , OPTIC DIAMETERS 9.5 - 10.5 , ZONAL CURVATURES ARE

NE NE 5.3 5.45 5.55 5.7 5.85 5.95 6.1 6.25 6.4 6.55 6.7 6.85 7 7.15 7.3 7.45 7.6

FOR EDGE LIFT 0.1 , OPTIC DIAMETERS 5 - 6 , ZONAL CURVATURES ARE

6.8 7.05 7.3 7.5 7.75 8.05 8.3 8.55 8.85 9.1 9.4 9.7 10 10.35 10.65 11 11.3 11.65 12.05

FOR EDGE LIFT 0.1 , OPTIC DIAMETERS 5.5 - 6.5 , ZONAL CURVATURES ARE

6.4 6.65 6.85 7.05 7.3 7.5 7.75 8 8.25 8.5 8.75 9 9.25 9.55 9.8 10.1 10.4 10.7 11

FOR EDGE LIFT 0.1 , OPTIC DIAMETERS 6 - 7 , ZONAL CURVATURES ARE

6.1 6.3 6.5 6.7 6.9 7.1 7.35 7.55 7.75 8 8.2 8.45 8.7 8.95 9.2 9.45 9.7 10 10.25

FOR EDGE LIFT 0.1 , OPTIC DIAMETERS 6.5 - 7.5 , ZONAL CURVATURES ARE

5.85 6.05 6.2 6.4 6.6 6.8 7 7.2 7.4 7.6 7.8 8 8.25 8.45 8.7 8.95 9.15 9.4 9.65

FOR EDGE LIFT 0.1 , OPTIC DIAMETERS 7 - 8 , ZONAL CURVATURES ARE

5.65 5.8 6 6.15 6.35 6.5 6.7 6.9 7.1 7.25 7.45 7.65 7.85 8.1 8.3 8.5 8.7 8.95 9.15

FOR EDGE LIFT 0.1 , OPTIC DIAMETERS 7.5 - 8.5 , ZONAL CURVATURES ARE

5.5 5.65 5.8 5.95 6.1 6.3 6.45 6.65 6.8 7 7.2 7.35 7.55 7.75 7.95 8.15 8.35 8.55 8.75

FOR EDGE LIFT 0.1 , OPTIC DIAMETERS 8 - 9 , ZONAL CURVATURES ARE

5.35 5.5 5.65 5.8 5.95 6.1 6.25 6.45 6.6 6.75 6.95 7.15 7.3 7.5 7.65 7.85 8.05 8.25 8.45

FOR EDGE LIFT 0.1 , OPTIC DIAMETERS 8.5 - 9.5 , ZONAL CURVATURES ARE

5.25 5.35 5.5 5.65 5.8 5.95 6.1 6.25 6.4 6.6 6.75 6.9 7.1 7.25 7.45 7.6 7.8 7.95 8.15

FOR EDGE LIFT 0.1 , OPTIC DIAMETERS 9 - 10 , ZONAL CURVATURES ARE

5.15 5.25 5.4 5.55 5.7 5.8 5.95 6.1 6.25 6.4 6.6 6.75 6.9 7.05 7.2 7.4 7.55 7.75 7.9

FOR EDGE LIFT 0.1 , OPTIC DIAMETERS 9.5 - 10.5 , ZONAL CURVATURES ARE

NE NE 5.3 5.45 5.6 5.7 5.85 6 6.15 6.3 6.45 6.6 6.75 6.9 7.05 7.2 7.35 7.55 7.7

```
FOR EDGE LIFT   0.11 ,   OPTIC DIAMETERS   5 - 6 ,   ZONAL CURVATURES ARE
 7.1  7.35  7.6  7.9  8.15  8.45  8.75  9.05  9.35  9.7  10  10.35  10.7  11.1  11.45  11.85  12.25  12.65  13.1

FOR EDGE LIFT   0.11 ,   OPTIC DIAMETERS   5.5 - 6.5 ,   ZONAL CURVATURES ARE
 6.6  6.85  7.1  7.3  7.55  7.8  8.1  8.35  8.6  8.9  9.2  9.5  9.8  10.1  10.4  10.75  11.1  11.45  11.8

FOR EDGE LIFT   0.11 ,   OPTIC DIAMETERS   6 - 7 ,   ZONAL CURVATURES ARE
 6.25  6.45  6.65  6.9  7.1  7.35  7.55  7.8  8.05  8.3  8.55  8.8  9.1  9.35  9.65  9.95  10.2  10.55  10.85

FOR EDGE LIFT   0.11 ,   OPTIC DIAMETERS   6.5 - 7.5 ,   ZONAL CURVATURES ARE
 5.95  6.15  6.35  6.55  6.75  6.95  7.15  7.4  7.6  7.85  8.05  8.3  8.55  8.8  9.05  9.3  9.55  9.85  10.1

FOR EDGE LIFT   0.11 ,   OPTIC DIAMETERS   7 - 8 ,   ZONAL CURVATURES ARE
 5.7  5.9  6.1  6.25  6.45  6.65  6.85  7.05  7.25  7.45  7.65  7.9  8.1  8.35  8.55  8.8  9.05  9.3  9.55

FOR EDGE LIFT   0.11 ,   OPTIC DIAMETERS   7.5 - 8.5 ,   ZONAL CURVATURES ARE
 5.5  5.7  5.85  6.05  6.2  6.4  6.55  6.75  6.95  7.15  7.35  7.55  7.75  7.95  8.15  8.4  8.6  8.85  9.05

FOR EDGE LIFT   0.11 ,   OPTIC DIAMETERS   8 - 9 ,   ZONAL CURVATURES ARE
 5.35  5.5  5.7  5.85  6  6.15  6.35  6.5  6.7  6.9  7.05  7.25  7.45  7.65  7.85  8.05  8.25  8.45  8.65

FOR EDGE LIFT   0.11 ,   OPTIC DIAMETERS   8.5 - 9.5 ,   ZONAL CURVATURES ARE
 5.25  5.4  5.55  5.7  5.85  6  6.15  6.3  6.5  6.65  6.85  7  7.2  7.35  7.55  7.75  7.95  8.15  8.35

FOR EDGE LIFT   0.11 ,   OPTIC DIAMETERS   9 - 10 ,   ZONAL CURVATURES ARE
 5.15  5.3  5.4  5.55  5.7  5.85  6  6.15  6.3  6.45  6.65  6.8  6.95  7.15  7.3  7.5  7.7  7.85  8.05

FOR EDGE LIFT   0.11 ,   OPTIC DIAMETERS   9.5 - 10.5 ,   ZONAL CURVATURES ARE
NE  NE  5.35  5.45  5.6  5.75  5.85  6  6.15  6.3  6.45  6.65  6.8  6.95  7.1  7.3  7.45  7.65  7.8
```

FOR EDGE LIFT 0.12 , OPTIC DIAMETERS 5 - 6 , ZONAL CURVATURES ARE

7.4 7.65 7.95 8.25 8.6 8.9 9.25 9.6 9.95 10.35 10.7 11.1 11.55 11.95 12.4 12.85 13.35 13.85 14.35

FOR EDGE LIFT 0.12 , OPTIC DIAMETERS 5.5 - 6.5 , ZONAL CURVATURES ARE

6.85 7.1 7.35 7.6 7.9 8.15 8.45 8.75 9.05 9.35 9.7 10.05 10.35 10.75 11.1 11.5 11.85 12.25 12.7

FOR EDGE LIFT 0.12 , OPTIC DIAMETERS 6 - 7 , ZONAL CURVATURES ARE

6.4 6.65 6.85 7.1 7.35 7.6 7.85 8.1 8.4 8.65 8.95 9.25 9.55 9.85 10.15 10.45 10.8 11.15 11.5

FOR EDGE LIFT 0.12 , OPTIC DIAMETERS 6.5 - 7.5 , ZONAL CURVATURES ARE

6.05 6.25 6.5 6.7 6.9 7.15 7.35 7.6 7.85 8.1 8.35 8.6 8.9 9.15 9.45 9.7 10 10.3 10.6

FOR EDGE LIFT 0.12 , OPTIC DIAMETERS 7 - 8 , ZONAL CURVATURES ARE

5.8 6 6.2 6.35 6.6 6.8 7 7.2 7.45 7.65 7.9 8.1 8.35 8.6 8.85 9.1 9.4 9.65 9.9

FOR EDGE LIFT 0.12 , OPTIC DIAMETERS 7.5 - 8.5 , ZONAL CURVATURES ARE

5.55 5.75 5.95 6.1 6.3 6.5 6.7 6.9 7.1 7.3 7.5 7.7 7.95 8.15 8.4 8.65 8.85 9.1 9.35

FOR EDGE LIFT 0.12 , OPTIC DIAMETERS 8 - 9 , ZONAL CURVATURES ARE

5.4 5.55 5.7 5.9 6.05 6.25 6.4 6.6 6.8 7 7.2 7.4 7.6 7.8 8 8.25 8.45 8.7 8.9

FOR EDGE LIFT 0.12 , OPTIC DIAMETERS 8.5 - 9.5 , ZONAL CURVATURES ARE

5.25 5.4 5.55 5.7 5.9 6.05 6.2 6.4 6.55 6.75 6.9 7.1 7.3 7.5 7.7 7.9 8.1 8.3 8.5

FOR EDGE LIFT 0.12 , OPTIC DIAMETERS 9 - 10 , ZONAL CURVATURES ARE

5.15 5.3 5.45 5.55 5.7 5.9 6.05 6.2 6.35 6.55 6.7 6.9 7.05 7.25 7.4 7.6 7.8 8 8.2

FOR EDGE LIFT 0.12 , OPTIC DIAMETERS 9.5 - 10.5 , ZONAL CURVATURES ARE

NE NE 5.35 5.45 5.6 5.75 5.9 6.05 6.2 6.35 6.5 6.7 6.85 7 7.2 7.35 7.55 7.75 7.9

```
FOR EDGE LIFT   0.13 ,   OPTIC DIAMETERS   5 - 6 ,   ZONAL CURVATURES ARE
 7.7  8.05  8.35  8.7  9.05  9.45  9.8  10.2  10.65  11.1  11.55  12  12.5  13  13.55  14.1  14.7  15.3  15.95

FOR EDGE LIFT   0.13 ,   OPTIC DIAMETERS   5.5 - 6.5 ,   ZONAL CURVATURES ARE
 7.05  7.35  7.6  7.9  8.2  8.55  8.85  9.2  9.55  9.9  10.25  10.65  11.05  11.45  11.9  12.35  12.8  13.25  13.75

FOR EDGE LIFT   0.13 ,   OPTIC DIAMETERS   6 - 7 ,   ZONAL CURVATURES ARE
 6.55  6.8  7.05  7.3  7.6  7.85  8.15  8.45  8.75  9.05  9.35  9.7  10  10.35  10.7  11.1  11.5  11.85  12.3

FOR EDGE LIFT   0.13 ,   OPTIC DIAMETERS   6.5 - 7.5 ,   ZONAL CURVATURES ARE
 6.2  6.4  6.65  6.85  7.1  7.35  7.6  7.85  8.1  8.4  8.65  8.95  9.25  9.55  9.85  10.2  10.5  10.85  11.2

FOR EDGE LIFT   0.13 ,   OPTIC DIAMETERS   7 - 8 ,   ZONAL CURVATURES ARE
 5.9  6.1  6.3  6.5  6.7  6.95  7.15  7.4  7.6  7.85  8.1  8.4  8.65  8.9  9.2  9.45  9.75  10.05  10.35

FOR EDGE LIFT   0.13 ,   OPTIC DIAMETERS   7.5 - 8.5 ,   ZONAL CURVATURES ARE
 5.65  5.8  6  6.2  6.4  6.6  6.8  7  7.25  7.45  7.7  7.9  8.15  8.4  8.65  8.9  9.15  9.45  9.7

FOR EDGE LIFT   0.13 ,   OPTIC DIAMETERS   8 - 9 ,   ZONAL CURVATURES ARE
 5.45  5.6  5.75  5.95  6.15  6.3  6.5  6.7  6.9  7.1  7.3  7.55  7.75  8  8.2  8.45  8.7  8.9  9.15

FOR EDGE LIFT   0.13 ,   OPTIC DIAMETERS   8.5 - 9.5 ,   ZONAL CURVATURES ARE
 5.25  5.45  5.6  5.75  5.9  6.1  6.25  6.45  6.65  6.8  7  7.2  7.4  7.65  7.85  8.05  8.25  8.5  8.75

FOR EDGE LIFT   0.13 ,   OPTIC DIAMETERS   9 - 10 ,   ZONAL CURVATURES ARE
 5.15  5.3  5.45  5.6  5.75  5.9  6.05  6.25  6.4  6.6  6.75  6.95  7.15  7.35  7.55  7.75  7.95  8.15  8.35

FOR EDGE LIFT   0.13 ,   OPTIC DIAMETERS   9.5 - 10.5 ,   ZONAL CURVATURES ARE
NE  NE   5.35  5.45  5.6  5.75  5.9  6.05  6.25  6.4  6.55  6.75  6.9  7.1  7.25  7.45  7.65  7.85  8.05
```

```
FOR EDGE LIFT   0.14 ,   OPTIC DIAMETERS   5 - 6 ,   ZONAL CURVATURES ARE
8.1 8.45 8.8 9.2 9.6 10.05 10.5 10.95 11.45 11.95 12.5 13.05 13.65 14.25 14.95 15.6 16.35 17.15 17.95

FOR EDGE LIFT   0.14 ,   OPTIC DIAMETERS   5.5 - 6.5 ,   ZONAL CURVATURES ARE
7.3 7.65 7.95 8.25 8.6 8.95 9.3 9.7 10.1 10.5 10.95 11.35 11.85 12.3 12.8 13.35 13.9 14.45 15.05

FOR EDGE LIFT   0.14 ,   OPTIC DIAMETERS   6 - 7 ,   ZONAL CURVATURES ARE
6.75 7 7.3 7.55 7.85 8.15 8.45 8.8 9.15 9.45 9.85 10.2 10.55 10.95 11.4 11.8 12.25 12.7 13.2

FOR EDGE LIFT   0.14 ,   OPTIC DIAMETERS   6.5 - 7.5 ,   ZONAL CURVATURES ARE
6.3 6.55 6.8 7.05 7.3 7.55 7.85 8.1 8.4 8.7 9 9.35 9.65 10 10.35 10.7 11.05 11.45 11.85

FOR EDGE LIFT   0.14 ,   OPTIC DIAMETERS   7 - 8 ,   ZONAL CURVATURES ARE
5.95 6.15 6.4 6.6 6.85 7.1 7.35 7.6 7.85 8.1 8.35 8.65 8.95 9.25 9.55 9.85 10.2 10.5 10.85

FOR EDGE LIFT   0.14 ,   OPTIC DIAMETERS   7.5 - 8.5 ,   ZONAL CURVATURES ARE
5.7 5.9 6.05 6.3 6.5 6.7 6.9 7.15 7.4 7.6 7.85 8.1 8.4 8.65 8.9 9.2 9.5 9.8 10.1

FOR EDGE LIFT   0.14 ,   OPTIC DIAMETERS   8 - 9 ,   ZONAL CURVATURES ARE
5.45 5.65 5.8 6 6.2 6.4 6.6 6.8 7 7.25 7.45 7.7 7.9 8.15 8.4 8.65 8.9 9.2 9.45

FOR EDGE LIFT   0.14 ,   OPTIC DIAMETERS   8.5 - 9.5 ,   ZONAL CURVATURES ARE
5.3 5.45 5.6 5.8 5.95 6.15 6.35 6.5 6.7 6.9 7.1 7.35 7.55 7.75 8 8.2 8.45 8.7 8.95

FOR EDGE LIFT   0.14 ,   OPTIC DIAMETERS   9 - 10 ,   ZONAL CURVATURES ARE
5.15 5.3 5.45 5.6 5.75 5.95 6.1 6.3 6.45 6.65 6.85 7.05 7.25 7.45 7.65 7.85 8.1 8.3 8.55

FOR EDGE LIFT   0.14 ,   OPTIC DIAMETERS   9.5 - 10.5 ,   ZONAL CURVATURES ARE
NE NE 5.35 5.5 5.65 5.8 5.95 6.1 6.25 6.45 6.6 6.8 6.95 7.15 7.35 7.55 7.75 7.95 8.15
```

```
FOR EDGE LIFT    0.15 ,    OPTIC DIAMETERS    5  -  6 ,     ZONAL CURVATURES ARE
 8.5  8.9  9.35  9.8  10.25  10.75  11.25  11.8  12.4  13  13.65  14.35  15.05  15.85  16.65  17.55  18.45  19.5  20.55

FOR EDGE LIFT    0.15 ,    OPTIC DIAMETERS    5.5  -  6.5 ,     ZONAL CURVATURES ARE
 7.6  7.95  8.3  8.65  9.05  9.45  9.85  10.25  10.7  11.2  11.7  12.2  12.75  13.3  13.9  14.55  15.2  15.9  16.65

FOR EDGE LIFT    0.15 ,    OPTIC DIAMETERS    6  -  7 ,     ZONAL CURVATURES ARE
 6.95  7.25  7.55  7.85  8.15  8.5  8.85  9.2  9.55  9.95  10.35  10.75  11.2  11.65  12.15  12.6  13.15  13.65  14.25

FOR EDGE LIFT    0.15 ,    OPTIC DIAMETERS    6.5  -  7.5 ,     ZONAL CURVATURES ARE
 6.45  6.7  6.95  7.25  7.5  7.8  8.1  8.4  8.7  9.05  9.4  9.75  10.1  10.5  10.9  11.3  11.7  12.15  12.6

FOR EDGE LIFT    0.15 ,    OPTIC DIAMETERS    7  -  8 ,     ZONAL CURVATURES ARE
 6.05  6.3  6.5  6.75  7  7.25  7.5  7.8  8.05  8.35  8.65  8.95  9.3  9.6  9.95  10.3  10.65  11  11.4

FOR EDGE LIFT    0.15 ,    OPTIC DIAMETERS    7.5  -  8.5 ,     ZONAL CURVATURES ARE
 5.75  5.95  6.15  6.35  6.6  6.8  7.05  7.3  7.55  7.8  8.05  8.35  8.65  8.9  9.2  9.5  9.85  10.15  10.5

FOR EDGE LIFT    0.15 ,    OPTIC DIAMETERS    8  -  9 ,     ZONAL CURVATURES ARE
 5.5  5.7  5.85  6.05  6.25  6.45  6.7  6.9  7.15  7.35  7.6  7.85  8.1  8.35  8.65  8.9  9.2  9.5  9.75

FOR EDGE LIFT    0.15 ,    OPTIC DIAMETERS    8.5  -  9.5 ,     ZONAL CURVATURES ARE
 5.3  5.45  5.65  5.8  6  6.2  6.4  6.6  6.8  7  7.25  7.45  7.7  7.9  8.15  8.4  8.65  8.9  9.2

FOR EDGE LIFT    0.15 ,    OPTIC DIAMETERS    9  -  10 ,     ZONAL CURVATURES ARE
 5.15  5.3  5.45  5.65  5.3  5.95  6.15  6.35  6.5  6.7  6.9  7.1  7.35  7.55  7.75  8  8.25  8.45  8.7

FOR EDGE LIFT    0.15 ,    OPTIC DIAMETERS    9.5  -  10.5 ,     ZONAL CURVATURES ARE
NE  NE   5.35  5.5  5.65  5.8  5.95  6.1  6.3  6.45  6.65  6.85  7.05  7.25  7.45  7.65  7.85  8.1  8.3
```

TABLE III **Back Peripheral Optic Radii (Zonal Curvatures) for the following:**
BCOR 7.0 to 8.8 in 0.1 steps
Zone Width 0.2 **Zone Inner Diameters** 7.0 to 10.6 in 0.2 steps
Axial Edge Lift Components 0.01 to 0.15 in 0.01 steps

FOR EDGE LIFT 0.01 , OPTIC DIAMETERS 7 - 7.4 , ZONAL CURVATURES ARE

7.45 7.6 7.7 7.85 7.95 8.1 8.2 8.35 8.45 8.6 8.7 8.85 8.95 9.1 9.2 9.35 9.45 9.6 9.75

FOR EDGE LIFT 0.01 , OPTIC DIAMETERS 7.2 - 7.6 , ZONAL CURVATURES ARE

7.45 7.55 7.7 7.8 7.95 8.05 8.2 8.3 8.4 8.55 8.65 8.8 8.9 9.05 9.2 9.3 9.45 9.55 9.7

FOR EDGE LIFT 0.01 , OPTIC DIAMETERS 7.4 - 7.8 , ZONAL CURVATURES ARE

7.4 7.55 7.65 7.8 7.9 8 8.15 8.25 8.4 8.5 8.65 8.75 8.9 9 9.15 9.25 9.4 9.5 9.65

FOR EDGE LIFT 0.01 , OPTIC DIAMETERS 7.6 - 8. , ZONAL CURVATURES ARE

7.4 7.5 7.65 7.75 7.85 8 8.1 8.25 8.35 8.5 8.6 8.75 8.85 9 9.1 9.25 9.35 9.5 9.6

FOR EDGE LIFT 0.01 , OPTIC DIAMETERS 7.8 - 8.2 , ZONAL CURVATURES ARE

7.35 7.5 7.6 7.75 7.85 7.95 8.1 8.2 8.35 8.45 8.55 8.7 8.8 8.95 9.05 9.2 9.3 9.45 9.55

FOR EDGE LIFT 0.01 , OPTIC DIAMETERS 8. - 8.4 , ZONAL CURVATURES ARE

7.35 7.45 7.6 7.7 7.8 7.95 8.05 8.2 8.3 8.4 8.55 8.65 8.8 8.9 9.05 9.15 9.3 9.4 9.55

FOR EDGE LIFT 0.01 , OPTIC DIAMETERS 8.2 - 8.6 , ZONAL CURVATURES ARE

7.3 7.45 7.55 7.7 7.8 7.9 8.05 8.15 8.3 8.4 8.5 8.65 8.75 8.9 9 9.15 9.25 9.35 9.5

FOR EDGE LIFT 0.01 , OPTIC DIAMETERS 8.4 - 8.8 , ZONAL CURVATURES ARE

7.3 7.4 7.55 7.65 7.75 7.9 8 8.15 8.25 8.35 8.5 8.6 8.75 8.85 8.95 9.1 9.2 9.35 9.45

FOR EDGE LIFT 0.01 , OPTIC DIAMETERS 8.6 - 9 , ZONAL CURVATURES ARE

7.3 7.4 7.5 7.65 7.75 7.85 8 8.1 8.2 8.35 8.45 8.6 8.7 8.8 8.95 9.05 9.2 9.3 9.45

FOR EDGE LIFT 0.01 , OPTIC DIAMETERS 8.8 - 9.2 , ZONAL CURVATURES ARE

7.25 7.4 7.5 7.6 7.75 7.85 7.95 8.1 8.2 8.3 8.45 8.55 8.7 8.8 8.9 9.05 9.15 9.3 9.4

FOR EDGE LIFT 0.01 , OPTIC DIAMETERS 9. - 9.4 , ZONAL CURVATURES ARE

7.25 7.35 7.5 7.6 7.7 7.85 7.95 8.05 8.2 8.3 8.4 8.55 8.65 8.75 8.9 9 9.15 9.25 9.35

FOR EDGE LIFT 0.01 , OPTIC DIAMETERS 9.2 - 9.6 , ZONAL CURVATURES ARE

7.25 7.35 7.45 7.55 7.7 7.8 7.9 8.05 8.15 8.25 8.4 8.5 8.65 8.75 8.85 9 9.1 9.25 9.35

FOR EDGE LIFT 0.01 , OPTIC DIAMETERS 9.4 - 9.8 , ZONAL CURVATURES ARE

7.2 7.3 7.45 7.55 7.65 7.8 7.9 8 8.15 8.25 8.35 8.5 8.6 8.7 8.85 8.95 9.1 9.2 9.3

FOR EDGE LIFT 0.01 , OPTIC DIAMETERS 9.6 - 10. , ZONAL CURVATURES ARE

7.2 7.3 7.4 7.55 7.65 7.75 7.9 8 8.1 8.25 8.35 8.45 8.6 8.7 8.8 8.95 9.05 9.2 9.3

FOR EDGE LIFT 0.01 , OPTIC DIAMETERS 9.8 - 10.2 , ZONAL CURVATURES ARE

7.2 7.3 7.4 7.5 7.65 7.75 7.85 8 8.1 8.2 8.35 3.45 8.55 8.7 8.8 8.9 9.05 9.15 9.25

FOR EDGE LIFT 0.01 , OPTIC DIAMETERS 10. - 10.4 , ZONAL CURVATURES ARE

7.15 7.3 7.4 7.5 7.6 7.75 7.85 7.95 8.1 8.2 8.3 8.45 8.55 8.65 8.8 8.9 9 9.15 9.25

FOR EDGE LIFT 0.01 , OPTIC DIAMETERS 10.2 - 10.6 , ZONAL CURVATURES ARE

7.15 7.25 7.4 7.5 7.6 7.7 7.85 7.95 8.05 8.15 8.3 8.4 8.5 8.65 8.75 8.85 9 9.1 9.2

FOR EDGE LIFT 0.01 , OPTIC DIAMETERS 10.4 - 10.8 , ZONAL CURVATURES ARE

7.15 7.25 7.35 7.45 7.6 7.7 7.8 7.95 8.05 8.15 8.25 8.4 8.5 8.6 8.75 8.85 8.95 9.1 9.2

FOR EDGE LIFT 0.01 , OPTIC DIAMETERS 10.6 - 11. , ZONAL CURVATURES ARE

7.1 7.25 7.35 7.45 7.55 7.7 7.8 7.9 8.05 8.15 8.25 8.35 8.5 8.6 8.7 8.85 8.95 9.05 9.2

```
FOR EDGE LIFT   0.02 ,   OPTIC DIAMETERS   7  -  7.4 ,   ZONAL CURVATURES ARE
 8.05  8.2  8.35  8.5  8.65  8.8  8.95  9.15  9.3  9.45  9.6  9.75  9.95  10.1  10.25  10.45  10.6  10.75  10.95

FOR EDGE LIFT   0.02 ,   OPTIC DIAMETERS   7.2  -  7.6 ,   ZONAL CURVATURES ARE
 8  8.15  8.3  8.45  8.6  8.75  8.9  9.05  9.2  9.35  9.5  9.7  9.85  10  10.15  10.35  10.5  10.65  10.85

FOR EDGE LIFT   0.02 ,   OPTIC DIAMETERS   7.4  -  7.8 ,   ZONAL CURVATURES ARE
 7.9  8.05  8.2  8.35  8.5  8.65  8.8  8.95  9.15  9.3  9.45  9.6  9.75  9.9  10.05  10.25  10.4  10.55  10.75

FOR EDGE LIFT   0.02 ,   OPTIC DIAMETERS   7.6  -  8. ,   ZONAL CURVATURES ARE
 7.85  8  8.15  8.3  8.45  8.6  8.75  8.9  9.05  9.2  9.35  9.5  9.65  9.85  10  10.15  10.3  10.45  10.65

FOR EDGE LIFT   0.02 ,   OPTIC DIAMETERS   7.8  -  8.2 ,   ZONAL CURVATURES ARE
 7.8  7.95  8.1  8.25  8.4  8.55  8.7  8.85  9  9.15  9.3  9.45  9.6  9.75  9.9  10.05  10.2  10.4  10.55

FOR EDGE LIFT   0.02 ,   OPTIC DIAMETERS   8.  -  8.4 ,   ZONAL CURVATURES ARE
 7.75  7.9  8.05  8.2  8.35  8.45  8.6  8.75  8.9  9.05  9.2  9.35  9.5  9.65  9.8  10  10.15  10.3  10.45

FOR EDGE LIFT   0.02 ,   OPTIC DIAMETERS   8.2  -  8.6 ,   ZONAL CURVATURES ARE
 7.7  7.85  8  8.15  8.25  8.4  8.55  8.7  8.85  9  9.15  9.3  9.45  9.6  9.75  9.9  10.05  10.2  10.35

FOR EDGE LIFT   0.02 ,   OPTIC DIAMETERS   8.4  -  8.8 ,   ZONAL CURVATURES ARE
 7.65  7.8  7.95  8.1  8.2  8.35  8.5  8.65  8.8  8.95  9.1  9.25  9.4  9.55  9.7  9.85  10  10.15  10.3

FOR EDGE LIFT   0.02 ,   OPTIC DIAMETERS   8.6  -  9 ,   ZONAL CURVATURES ARE
 7.6  7.75  7.9  8.05  8.15  8.3  8.45  8.6  8.75  8.9  9  9.15  9.3  9.45  9.6  9.75  9.9  10.05  10.2
```

FOR EDGE LIFT 0.02 , OPTIC DIAMETERS 8.8 - 9.2 , ZONAL CURVATURES ARE

7.55 7.7 7.85 8 8.1 8.25 8.4 8.55 8.7 8.8 8.95 9.1 9.25 9.4 9.55 9.7 9.85 10 10.15

FOR EDGE LIFT 0.02 , CPTIC DIAMETERS 9. - 9.4 , ZONAL CURVATURES ARE

7.55 7.65 7.8 7.95 8.05 8.2 8.35 8.5 8.65 8.75 8.9 9.05 9.2 9.35 9.5 9.65 9.8 9.95 10.05

FOR EDGE LIFT 0.02 , OPTIC DIAMETERS 9.2 - 9.6 , ZONAL CURVATURES ARE

7.5 7.6 7.75 7.9 8.05 8.15 8.3 8.45 8.6 8.7 8.85 9 9.15 9.3 9.45 9.55 9.7 9.85 10

FOR EDGE LIFT 0.02 , OPTIC DIAMETERS 9.4 - 9.8 , ZONAL CURVATURES ARE

7.45 7.6 7.7 7.85 8 3.1 8.25 8.4 8.55 8.65 8.8 8.95 9.1 9.25 9.35 9.5 9.65 9.8 9.95

FOR EDGE LIFT 0.02 , OPTIC DIAMETERS 9.6 - 10. , ZONAL CURVATURES ARE

7.4 7.55 7.7 7.8 7.95 8.1 8.2 8.35 8.5 8.6 8.75 8.9 9.05 9.2 9.3 9.45 9.6 9.75 9.9

FOR EDGE LIFT 0.02 , OPTIC DIAMETERS 9.8 - 10.2 , ZONAL CURVATURES ARE

7.4 7.5 7.65 7.75 7.9 8.05 8.15 8.3 8.45 8.6 8.7 8.85 9 9.15 9.25 9.4 9.55 9.7 9.85

FOR EDGE LIFT 0.02 , OPTIC DIAMETERS 10. - 10.4 , ZONAL CURVATURES ARE

7.35 7.5 7.6 7.75 7.85 8 8.15 8.25 8.4 8.55 8.65 8.8 8.95 9.1 9.2 9.35 9.5 9.65 9.8

FOR EDGE LIFT 0.02 , OPTIC DIAMETERS 10.2 - 10.6 , ZONAL CURVATURES ARE

7.3 7.45 7.55 7.7 7.85 7.95 8.1 8.25 8.35 8.5 8.65 8.75 8.9 9.05 9.15 9.3 9.45 9.6 9.75

FOR EDGE LIFT 0.02 , OPTIC DIAMETERS 10.4 - 10.8 , ZONAL CURVATURES ARE

7.3 7.4 7.55 7.65 7.8 7.95 8.05 8.2 8.3 8.45 8.6 8.7 8.85 9 9.15 9.25 9.4 9.55 9.7

FOR EDGE LIFT 0.02 , OPTIC DIAMETERS 10.6 - 11. , ZONAL CURVATURES ARE

7.25 7.4 7.5 7.65 7.75 7.9 8 8.15 8.3 8.4 8.55 8.7 8.8 8.95 9.1 9.2 9.35 9.5 9.65

```
FOR EDGE LIFT   0.03 ,   OPTIC DIAMETERS   7 - 7.4 ,   ZONAL CURVATURES ARE
 8.8  8.95  9.15  9.35  9.55  9.75  9.95  10.15  10.35  10.6  10.8  11  11.2  11.45  11.65  11.9  12.1  12.35  12.6

FOR EDGE LIFT   0.03 ,   OPTIC DIAMETERS   7.2 - 7.6 ,   ZONAL CURVATURES ARE
 8.65  8.85  9.05  9.2  9.4  9.6  9.8  10  10.2  10.4  10.6  10.85  11.05  11.25  11.45  11.7  11.9  12.15  12.35

FOR EDGE LIFT   0.03 ,   OPTIC DIAMETERS   7.4 - 7.8 ,   ZONAL CURVATURES ARE
 8.55  8.75  8.9  9.1  9.3  9.5  9.65  9.85  10.05  10.25  10.45  10.65  10.85  11.1  11.3  11.5  11.7  11.95  12.15

FOR EDGE LIFT   0.03 ,   OPTIC DIAMETERS   7.6 - 8. ,   ZONAL CURVATURES ARE
 8.45  8.6  8.8  9  9.15  9.35  9.55  9.75  9.9  10.1  10.3  10.5  10.7  10.9  11.15  11.35  11.55  11.75  12

FOR EDGE LIFT   0.03 ,   OPTIC DIAMETERS   7.8 - 8.2 ,   ZONAL CURVATURES ARE
 8.35  8.5  8.7  8.85  9.05  9.25  9.4  9.6  9.8  10  10.2  10.35  10.55  10.75  10.95  11.15  11.4  11.6  11.8

FOR EDGE LIFT   0.03 ,   OPTIC DIAMETERS   8. - 8.4 ,   ZONAL CURVATURES ARE
 8.25  8.4  8.6  8.75  8.95  9.15  9.3  9.5  9.65  9.85  10.05  10.25  10.45  10.65  10.8  11  11.2  11.45  11.65

FOR EDGE LIFT   0.03 ,   OPTIC DIAMETERS   8.2 - 8.6 ,   ZONAL CURVATURES ARE
 8.15  8.35  8.5  8.65  8.85  9  9.2  9.4  9.55  9.75  9.95  10.1  10.3  10.5  10.7  10.9  11.1  11.3  11.5

FOR EDGE LIFT   0.03 ,   OPTIC DIAMETERS   8.4 - 8.8 ,   ZONAL CURVATURES ARE
 8.1  8.25  8.4  8.6  8.75  8.9  9.1  9.25  9.45  9.65  9.8  10  10.2  10.35  10.55  10.75  10.95  11.15  11.35

FOR EDGE LIFT   0.03 ,   OPTIC DIAMETERS   8.6 - 9 ,   ZONAL CURVATURES ARE
 8  8.15  8.35  8.5  8.65  8.85  9  9.2  9.35  9.55  9.7  9.9  10.05  10.25  10.45  10.6  10.8  11  11.2
```

FOR EDGE LIFT 0.03 , OPTIC DIAMETERS 8.8 - 9.2 , ZONAL CURVATURES ARE

7.95 8.1 8.25 8.4 8.6 8.75 8.9 9.1 9.25 9.45 9.6 9.8 9.95 10.15 10.3 10.5 10.7 10.9 11.05

FOR EDGE LIFT 0.03 , OPTIC DIAMETERS 9. - 9.4 , ZONAL CURVATURES ARE

7.85 8 8.2 8.35 8.5 8.65 8.85 9 9.15 9.35 9.5 9.7 9.85 10.05 10.2 10.4 10.55 10.75 10.95

FOR EDGE LIFT 0.03 , OPTIC DIAMETERS 9.2 - 9.6 , ZONAL CURVATURES ARE

7.8 7.95 8.1 8.25 8.4 8.6 8.75 8.9 9.1 9.25 9.4 9.6 9.75 9.95 10.1 10.3 10.45 10.65 10.85

FOR EDGE LIFT 0.03 , OPTIC DIAMETERS 9.4 - 9.8 , ZONAL CURVATURES ARE

7.75 7.9 8.05 8.2 8.35 8.5 8.65 8.85 9 9.15 9.35 9.5 9.65 9.85 10 10.2 10.35 10.55 10.7

FOR EDGE LIFT 0.03 , OPTIC DIAMETERS 9.6 - 10. , ZONAL CURVATURES ARE

7.65 7.8 7.95 8.15 8.3 8.45 8.6 8.75 8.9 9.1 9.25 9.4 9.6 9.75 9.9 10.1 10.25 10.45 10.6

FOR EDGE LIFT 0.03 , OPTIC DIAMETERS 9.8 - 10.2 , ZONAL CURVATURES ARE

7.6 7.75 7.9 8.05 8.2 8.35 8.55 8.7 8.35 9 9.15 9.35 9.5 9.65 9.85 10 10.15 10.35 10.5

FOR EDGE LIFT 0.03 , OPTIC DIAMETERS 10. - 10.4 , ZONAL CURVATURES ARE

7.55 7.7 7.85 8 8.15 8.3 8.45 8.6 8.75 8.95 9.1 9.25 9.4 9.6 9.75 9.9 10.1 10.25 10.4

FOR EDGE LIFT 0.03 , OPTIC DIAMETERS 10.2 - 10.6 , ZONAL CURVATURES ARE

7.5 7.65 7.8 7.95 8.1 8.25 8.4 8.55 8.7 8.85 9 9.2 9.35 9.5 9.65 9.85 10 10.15 10.35

FOR EDGE LIFT 0.03 , OPTIC DIAMETERS 10.4 - 10.8 , ZONAL CURVATURES ARE

7.45 7.6 7.75 7.9 8.05 8.2 8.35 8.5 8.65 8.8 8.95 9.1 9.25 9.45 9.6 9.75 9.9 10.1 10.25

FOR EDGE LIFT 0.03 , OPTIC DIAMETERS 10.6 - 11. , ZONAL CURVATURES ARE

7.4 7.55 7.7 7.85 8 8.15 8.3 8.45 8.6 8.75 8.9 9.05 9.2 9.35 9.5 9.65 9.85 10 10.15

```
FOR EDGE LIFT   0.04 ,   OPTIC DIAMETERS   7 - 7.4 ,   ZONAL CURVATURES ARE
9.7  9.95  10.2  10.45  10.7  11  11.25  11.5  11.8  12.1  12.4  12.7  13  13.3  13.6  13.95  14.25  14.6  14.95

FOR EDGE LIFT   0.04 ,   OPTIC DIAMETERS   7.2 - 7.6 ,   ZONAL CURVATURES ARE
9.5  9.75  10  10.25  10.5  10.75  11  11.25  11.55  11.8  12.1  12.35  12.65  12.95  13.25  13.55  13.9  14.2  14.5

FOR EDGE LIFT   0.04 ,   OPTIC DIAMETERS   7.4 - 7.8 ,   ZONAL CURVATURES ARE
9.3  9.55  9.8  10  10.25  10.5  10.75  11  11.3  11.55  11.8  12.1  12.35  12.65  12.95  13.25  13.55  13.85  14.15

FOR EDGE LIFT   0.04 ,   OPTIC DIAMETERS   7.6 - 8. ,   ZONAL CURVATURES ARE
9.15  9.4  9.6  9.85  10.05  10.3  10.55  10.8  11.05  11.3  11.55  11.8  12.1  12.35  12.65  12.95  13.2  13.5  13.8

FOR EDGE LIFT   0.04 ,   OPTIC DIAMETERS   7.8 - 8.2 ,   ZONAL CURVATURES ARE
9  9.2  9.45  9.65  9.9  10.1  10.35  10.6  10.85  11.1  11.35  11.6  11.85  12.1  12.35  12.65  12.95  13.2  13.5

FOR EDGE LIFT   0.04 ,   OPTIC DIAMETERS   8. - 8.4 ,   ZONAL CURVATURES ARE
8.85  9.05  9.25  9.5  9.7  9.95  10.15  10.4  10.65  10.85  11.1  11.35  11.6  11.85  12.15  12.4  12.65  12.95  13.2

FOR EDGE LIFT   0.04 ,   OPTIC DIAMETERS   8.2 - 8.6 ,   ZONAL CURVATURES ARE
8.7  8.9  9.15  9.35  9.55  9.75  10  10.2  10.45  10.7  10.9  11.15  11.4  11.65  11.9  12.15  12.4  12.65  12.95

FOR EDGE LIFT   0.04 ,   OPTIC DIAMETERS   8.4 - 8.8 ,   ZONAL CURVATURES ARE
8.6  8.8  9  9.2  9.4  9.6  9.85  10.05  10.25  10.5  10.75  10.95  11.2  11.45  11.7  11.95  12.2  12.45  12.7

FOR EDGE LIFT   0.04 ,   OPTIC DIAMETERS   8.6 - 9 ,   ZONAL CURVATURES ARE
8.45  8.65  8.85  9.05  9.25  9.45  9.7  9.9  10.1  10.35  10.55  10.8  11  11.25  11.5  11.7  11.95  12.2  12.45
```

```
FOR EDGE LIFT   0.04 ,   OPTIC DIAMETERS   8.8  -  9.2 ,   ZONAL CURVATURES ARE
 8.35  8.55  8.75  8.95  9.15  9.35  9.55  9.75  9.95  10.15  10.4  10.6  10.85  11.05  11.3  11.55  11.75  12  12.25

FOR EDGE LIFT   0.04 ,   OPTIC DIAMETERS   9.  -  9.4 ,   ZONAL CURVATURES ARE
 8.25  8.45  8.6  8.8  9  9.2  9.4  9.6  9.8  10.05  10.25  10.45  10.65  10.9  11.1  11.35  11.55  11.8  12.05

FOR EDGE LIFT   0.04 ,   OPTIC DIAMETERS   9.2  -  9.6 ,   ZONAL CURVATURES ARE
 8.15  8.35  8.5  8.7  8.9  9.1  9.3  9.5  9.7  9.9  10.1  10.3  10.5  10.75  10.95  11.15  11.4  11.65  11.85

FOR EDGE LIFT   0.04 ,   OPTIC DIAMETERS   9.4  -  9.8 ,   ZONAL CURVATURES ARE
 8.05  8.25  8.4  8.6  8.8  8.95  9.15  9.35  9.55  9.75  9.95  10.15  10.35  10.6  10.8  11  11.25  11.45  11.7

FOR EDGE LIFT   0.04 ,   OPTIC DIAMETERS   9.6  -  10. ,   ZONAL CURVATURES ARE
 7.95  8.15  8.3  8.5  8.7  8.85  9.05  9.25  9.45  9.65  9.85  10.05  10.25  10.45  10.65  10.85  11.05  11.3  11.5

FOR EDGE LIFT   0.04 ,   OPTIC DIAMETERS   9.8  -  10.2 ,   ZONAL CURVATURES ARE
 7.9  8.05  8.25  8.4  8.6  8.75  8.95  9.15  9.3  9.5  9.7  9.9  10.1  10.3  10.5  10.7  10.95  11.15  11.35

FOR EDGE LIFT   0.04 ,   OPTIC DIAMETERS   10.  -  10.4 ,   ZONAL CURVATURES ARE
 7.8  7.95  8.15  8.3  8.5  8.65  8.85  9.05  9.2  9.4  9.6  9.8  10  10.2  10.4  10.6  10.8  11  11.2

FOR EDGE LIFT   0.04 ,   OPTIC DIAMETERS   10.2  -  10.6 ,   ZONAL CURVATURES ARE
 7.75  7.9  8.05  8.25  8.4  8.6  8.75  8.95  9.1  9.3  9.5  9.65  9.85  10.05  10.25  10.45  10.65  10.85  11.05

FOR EDGE LIFT   0.04 ,   OPTIC DIAMETERS   10.4  -  10.8 ,   ZONAL CURVATURES ARE
 7.65  7.8  8  8.15  8.3  8.5  8.65  8.85  9  9.2  9.4  9.55  9.75  9.95  10.15  10.35  10.55  10.75  10.95

FOR EDGE LIFT   0.04 ,   OPTIC DIAMETERS   10.6  -  11. ,   ZONAL CURVATURES ARE
 7.6  7.75  7.9  8.05  8.25  8.4  8.6  8.75  8.95  9.1  9.3  9.45  9.65  9.85  10  10.2  10.4  10.6  10.8
```

```
FOR EDGE LIFT   0.05 ,   OPTIC DIAMETERS   7 - 7.4 ,   ZONAL CURVATURES ARE
 10.9  11.25  11.55  11.9  12.25  12.65  13  13.4  13.8  14.2  14.65  15.05  15.5  15.95  16.45  16.95  17.45  17.95  18.5

FOR EDGE LIFT   0.05 ,   OPTIC DIAMETERS   7.2 - 7.6 ,   ZONAL CURVATURES ARE
 10.6  10.9  11.25  11.55  11.9  12.25  12.6  12.95  13.35  13.7  14.1  14.5  14.95  15.35  15.8  16.25  16.75  17.2  17.75

FOR EDGE LIFT   0.05 ,   OPTIC DIAMETERS   7.4 - 7.8 ,   ZONAL CURVATURES ARE
 10.3  10.6  10.9  11.25  11.55  11.85  12.2  12.55  12.9  13.3  13.65  14.05  14.45  14.85  15.25  15.7  16.1  16.55  17.05

FOR EDGE LIFT   0.05 ,   OPTIC DIAMETERS   7.6 - 8. ,   ZONAL CURVATURES ARE
 10.05  10.35  10.65  10.95  11.25  11.55  11.85  12.2  12.55  12.9  13.25  13.6  13.95  14.35  14.75  15.15  15.55  16  16.45

FOR EDGE LIFT   0.05 ,   OPTIC DIAMETERS   7.8 - 8.2 ,   ZONAL CURVATURES ARE
 9.8  10.1  10.35  10.65  10.95  11.25  11.55  11.85  12.2  12.5  12.85  13.2  13.55  13.9  14.3  14.65  15.05  15.45  15.9

FOR EDGE LIFT   0.05 ,   OPTIC DIAMETERS   8. - 8.4 ,   ZONAL CURVATURES ARE
 9.6  9.85  10.15  10.4  10.7  10.95  11.25  11.55  11.85  12.2  12.5  12.85  13.2  13.5  13.9  14.25  14.6  15  15.4

FOR EDGE LIFT   0.05 ,   OPTIC DIAMETERS   8.2 - 8.6 ,   ZONAL CURVATURES ARE
 9.4  9.65  9.9  10.15  10.45  10.7  11  11.3  11.6  11.9  12.2  12.5  12.85  13.15  13.5  13.85  14.2  14.55  14.95

FOR EDGE LIFT   0.05 ,   OPTIC DIAMETERS   8.4 - 8.8 ,   ZONAL CURVATURES ARE
 9.2  9.45  9.7  9.95  10.2  10.5  10.75  11.05  11.3  11.6  11.9  12.2  12.5  12.85  13.15  13.5  13.8  14.15  14.5

FOR EDGE LIFT   0.05 ,   OPTIC DIAMETERS   8.6 - 9 ,   ZONAL CURVATURES ARE
 9.05  9.25  9.5  9.75  10  10.25  10.55  10.8  11.05  11.35  11.65  11.9  12.2  12.5  12.85  13.15  13.45  13.8  14.15
```

FOR EDGE LIFT 0.05 , OPTIC DIAMETERS 8.8 - 9.2 , ZONAL CURVATURES ARE

8.85 9.1 9.35 9.55 9.3 10.05 10.3 10.55 10.85 11.1 11.4 11.65 11.95 12.25 12.55 12.85 13.15 13.45 13.8

FOR EDGE LIFT 0.05 , OPTIC DIAMETERS 9. - 9.4 , ZONAL CURVATURES ARE

8.7 8.95 9.15 9.4 9.65 9.85 10.1 10.35 10.6 10.9 11.15 11.4 11.7 12 12.25 12.55 12.85 13.15 13.45

FOR EDGE LIFT 0.05 , OPTIC DIAMETERS 9.2 - 9.6 , ZONAL CURVATURES ARE

8.55 8.8 9 9.25 9.45 9.7 9.95 10.2 10.4 10.7 10.95 11.2 11.45 11.75 12 12.3 12.6 12.9 13.2

FOR EDGE LIFT 0.05 , OPTIC DIAMETERS 9.4 - 9.8 , ZONAL CURVATURES ARE

8.45 8.65 8.85 9.1 9.3 9.55 9.75 10 10.25 10.5 10.75 11 11.25 11.5 11.8 12.05 12.35 12.6 12.9

FOR EDGE LIFT 0.05 , OPTIC DIAMETERS 9.6 - 10. , ZONAL CURVATURES ARE

8.3 8.5 8.7 8.95 9.15 9.35 9.6 9.85 10.05 10.3 10.55 10.8 11.05 11.3 11.55 11.8 12.1 12.35 12.65

FOR EDGE LIFT 0.05 , OPTIC DIAMETERS 9.8 - 10.2 , ZONAL CURVATURES ARE

8.2 8.4 8.6 8.8 9 9.25 9.45 9.65 9.9 10.15 10.35 10.6 10.85 11.1 11.35 11.6 11.85 12.15 12.4

FOR EDGE LIFT 0.05 , OPTIC DIAMETERS 10. - 10.4 , ZONAL CURVATURES ARE

8.1 8.25 8.45 8.7 8.9 9.1 9.3 9.5 9.75 9.95 10.2 10.45 10.65 10.9 11.15 11.4 11.65 11.9 12.2

FOR EDGE LIFT 0.05 , OPTIC DIAMETERS 10.2 - 10.6 , ZONAL CURVATURES ARE

7.95 8.15 8.35 8.55 8.75 8.95 9.15 9.4 9.6 9.8 10.05 10.25 10.5 10.75 10.95 11.2 11.45 11.7 11.95

FOR EDGE LIFT 0.05 , OPTIC DIAMETERS 10.4 - 10.8 , ZONAL CURVATURES ARE

7.9 8.05 8.25 8.45 8.65 8.85 9.05 9.25 9.45 9.65 9.9 10.1 10.35 10.55 10.8 11.05 11.25 11.5 11.75

FOR EDGE LIFT 0.05 , OPTIC DIAMETERS 10.6 - 11. , ZONAL CURVATURES ARE

7.8 7.95 8.15 8.35 8.55 8.75 8.9 9.15 9.35 9.55 9.75 9.95 10.2 10.4 10.65 10.85 11.1 11.35 11.6

FOR EDGE LIFT 0.06 , OPTIC DIAMETERS 7 - 7.4 , ZONAL CURVATURES ARE

12.55 13 13.45 13.95 14.45 15 15.55 16.15 16.75 17.35 18 18.7 19.4 20.15 20.95 21.8 22.65 23.55 24.55

FOR EDGE LIFT 0.06 , OPTIC DIAMETERS 7.2 - 7.6 , ZONAL CURVATURES ARE

12.05 12.45 12.9 13.35 13.85 14.35 14.85 15.35 15.9 16.5 17.1 17.7 18.35 19.05 19.75 20.5 21.25 22.1 22.95

FOR EDGE LIFT 0.06 , OPTIC DIAMETERS 7.4 - 7.8 , ZONAL CURVATURES ARE

11.6 12 12.4 12.85 13.3 13.75 14.2 14.7 15.2 15.75 16.3 16.85 17.45 18.1 18.7 19.4 20.1 20.8 21.6

FOR EDGE LIFT 0.06 , OPTIC DIAMETERS 7.6 - 8. , ZONAL CURVATURES ARE

11.2 11.6 11.95 12.35 12.8 13.2 13.65 14.1 14.6 15.1 15.6 16.1 16.65 17.25 17.8 18.45 19.1 19.75 20.45

FOR EDGE LIFT 0.06 , OPTIC DIAMETERS 7.8 - 8.2 , ZONAL CURVATURES ARE

10.85 11.2 11.55 11.95 12.35 12.75 13.15 13.6 14.05 14.5 14.95 15.45 15.95 16.5 17.05 17.6 18.2 18.8 19.45

FOR EDGE LIFT 0.06 , OPTIC DIAMETERS 8. - 8.4 , ZONAL CURVATURES ARE

10.55 10.85 11.2 11.55 11.95 12.3 12.7 13.1 13.55 13.95 14.4 14.85 15.35 15.85 16.35 16.85 17.4 17.95 18.55

FOR EDGE LIFT 0.06 , OPTIC DIAMETERS 8.2 - 8.6 , ZONAL CURVATURES ARE

10.25 10.55 10.9 11.2 11.55 11.95 12.3 12.7 13.1 13.5 13.9 14.35 14.8 15.25 15.7 16.2 16.7 17.25 17.75

FOR EDGE LIFT 0.06 , OPTIC DIAMETERS 8.4 - 8.8 , ZONAL CURVATURES ARE

9.95 10.25 10.6 10.9 11.25 11.6 11.95 12.3 12.65 13.05 13.45 13.85 14.25 14.7 15.15 15.6 16.1 16.6 17.1

FOR EDGE LIFT 0.06 , OPTIC DIAMETERS 8.6 - 9 , ZONAL CURVATURES ARE

9.7 10 10.3 10.6 10.95 11.25 11.6 11.95 12.3 12.65 13.05 13.4 13.8 14.2 14.65 15.1 15.5 16 16.45

FOR EDGE LIFT 0.06 , OPTIC DIAMETERS 8.8 - 9.2 , ZONAL CURVATURES ARE

9.5 9.75 10.05 10.35 10.65 10.95 11.3 11.6 11.95 12.3 12.65 13 13.4 13.8 14.2 14.6 15 15.45 15.9

FOR EDGE LIFT 0.06 , OPTIC DIAMETERS 9. - 9.4 , ZONAL CURVATURES ARE

9.25 9.55 9.8 10.1 10.4 10.7 11 11.3 11.65 11.95 12.3 12.65 13 13.4 13.75 14.15 14.55 14.95 15.4

FOR EDGE LIFT 0.06 , OPTIC DIAMETERS 9.2 - 9.6 , ZONAL CURVATURES ARE

9.05 9.35 9.6 9.85 10.15 10.45 10.75 11.05 11.35 11.65 12 12.3 12.65 13 13.4 13.75 14.15 14.5 14.9

FOR EDGE LIFT 0.06 , OPTIC DIAMETERS 9.4 - 9.8 , ZONAL CURVATURES ARE

8.9 9.15 9.4 9.65 9.95 10.2 10.5 10.8 11.1 11.4 11.7 12 12.35 12.7 13.05 13.4 13.75 14.1 14.5

FOR EDGE LIFT 0.06 , OPTIC DIAMETERS 9.6 - 10. , ZONAL CURVATURES ARE

8.7 8.95 9.2 9.45 9.7 10 10.25 10.55 10.85 11.1 11.4 11.75 12.05 12.35 12.7 13.05 13.4 13.75 14.1

FOR EDGE LIFT 0.06 , OPTIC DIAMETERS 9.8 - 10.2 , ZONAL CURVATURES ARE

8.55 8.8 9.05 9.25 9.5 9.8 10.05 10.3 10.6 10.9 11.15 11.45 11.75 12.1 12.4 12.7 13.05 13.4 13.75

FOR EDGE LIFT 0.06 , OPTIC DIAMETERS 10. - 10.4 , ZONAL CURVATURES ARE

8.4 8.65 8.85 9.1 9.35 9.6 9.85 10.1 10.4 10.65 10.95 11.2 11.5 11.8 12.1 12.45 12.75 13.05 13.4

FOR EDGE LIFT 0.06 , OPTIC DIAMETERS 10.2 - 10.6 , ZONAL CURVATURES ARE

8.25 8.5 8.7 8.95 9.15 9.4 9.65 9.9 10.15 10.45 10.7 11 11.25 11.55 11.85 12.15 12.45 12.8 13.1

FOR EDGE LIFT 0.06 , OPTIC DIAMETERS 10.4 - 10.8 , ZONAL CURVATURES ARE

8.15 8.35 8.55 8.8 9 9.25 9.5 9.75 10 10.25 10.5 10.75 11.05 11.3 11.6 11.9 12.2 12.5 12.8

FOR EDGE LIFT 0.06 , OPTIC DIAMETERS 10.6 - 11. , ZONAL CURVATURES ARE

8 8.2 8.45 8.65 8.85 9.1 9.35 9.55 9.8 10.05 10.3 10.55 10.85 11.1 11.35 11.65 11.95 12.25 12.55

```
FOR EDGE LIFT   0.07 ,   OPTIC DIAMETERS   7  -  7.4 ,    ZONAL CURVATURES ARE
 14.85  15.55  16.25  17  17.75  18.6  19.5  20.45  21.45  22.5  23.65  24.9  26.2  27.65  29.15  30.85  32.65  34.6  36.8

FOR EDGE LIFT   0.07 ,   OPTIC DIAMETERS   7.2  -  7.6 ,    ZONAL CURVATURES ARE
 14.05  14.65  15.3  16  16.7  17.45  18.2  19.05  19.95  20.85  21.85  22.9  24.05  25.25  26.55  27.95  29.45  31.05  32.8

FOR EDGE LIFT   0.07 ,   OPTIC DIAMETERS   7.4  -  7.8 ,    ZONAL CURVATURES ARE
 13.35  13.9  14.5  15.1  15.75  16.45  17.15  17.9  18.65  19.5  20.35  21.3  22.3  23.35  24.45  25.65  26.9  28.3  29.75

FOR EDGE LIFT   0.07 ,   OPTIC DIAMETERS   7.6  -  8. ,    ZONAL CURVATURES ARE
 12.75  13.25  13.8  14.35  14.95  15.55  16.2  16.9  17.6  18.35  19.1  19.95  20.8  21.75  22.7  23.75  24.85  26.05  27.3

FOR EDGE LIFT   0.07 ,   OPTIC DIAMETERS   7.8  -  8.2 ,    ZONAL CURVATURES ARE
 12.2  12.7  13.2  13.7  14.25  14.8  15.4  16  16.65  17.35  18.05  18.8  19.55  20.4  21.25  22.15  23.15  24.15  25.25

FOR EDGE LIFT   0.07 ,   OPTIC DIAMETERS   8.  -  8.4 ,    ZONAL CURVATURES ARE
 11.75  12.2  12.65  13.1  13.6  14.15  14.7  15.25  15.85  16.45  17.1  17.8  18.5  19.25  20  20.85  21.7  22.6  23.55

FOR EDGE LIFT   0.07 ,   OPTIC DIAMETERS   8.2  -  8.6 ,    ZONAL CURVATURES ARE
 11.3  11.7  12.15  12.6  13.05  13.55  14.05  14.6  15.1  15.7  16.3  16.9  17.55  18.25  18.95  19.7  20.45  21.3  22.15

FOR EDGE LIFT   0.07 ,   OPTIC DIAMETERS   8.4  -  8.8 ,    ZONAL CURVATURES ARE
 10.9  11.3  11.7  12.15  12.55  13  13.5  14  14.5  15  15.55  16.15  16.75  17.35  18  18.7  19.4  20.15  20.9

FOR EDGE LIFT   0.07 ,   OPTIC DIAMETERS   8.6  -  9 ,    ZONAL CURVATURES ARE
 10.55  10.95  11.3  11.7  12.1  12.55  13  13.45  13.9  14.4  14.9  15.45  16  16.6  17.2  17.8  18.45  19.15  19.85
```

```
FOR EDGE LIFT   0.07 ,   OPTIC DIAMETERS   8.8  -  9.2 ,   ZONAL CURVATURES ARE
 10.25  10.6  10.95  11.3  11.7  12.1  12.55  12.95  13.4  13.85  14.35  14.85  15.35  15.9  16.45  17  17.6  18.25  18.9

FOR EDGE LIFT   0.07 ,   OPTIC DIAMETERS   9.  -  9.4 ,   ZONAL CURVATURES ARE
 9.95  10.25  10.6  10.95  11.35  11.7  12.1  12.5  12.95  13.35  13.8  14.3  14.75  15.25  15.8  16.35  16.9  17.45  18.05

FOR EDGE LIFT   0.07 ,   OPTIC DIAMETERS   9.2  -  9.6 ,   ZONAL CURVATURES ARE
 9.65  10  10.3  10.65  11  11.35  11.75  12.1  12.5  12.95  13.35  13.8  14.25  14.7  15.2  15.7  16.2  16.75  17.35

FOR EDGE LIFT   0.07 ,   OPTIC DIAMETERS   9.4  -  9.8 ,   ZONAL CURVATURES ARE
 9.4  9.7  10.05  10.35  10.7  11.05  11.4  11.75  12.15  12.5  12.9  13.35  13.75  14.2  14.65  15.15  15.65  16.15  16.65

FOR EDGE LIFT   0.07 ,   OPTIC DIAMETERS   9.6  -  10. ,   ZONAL CURVATURES ARE
 9.2  9.5  9.8  10.1  10.4  10.75  11.05  11.4  11.8  12.15  12.55  12.9  13.35  13.75  14.2  14.65  15.1  15.55  16.05

FOR EDGE LIFT   0.07 ,   OPTIC DIAMETERS   9.8  -  10.2 ,   ZONAL CURVATURES ARE
 8.95  9.25  9.55  9.85  10.15  10.45  10.8  11.1  11.45  11.8  12.15  12.55  12.95  13.3  13.75  14.15  14.6  15.05  15.5

FOR EDGE LIFT   0.07 ,   OPTIC DIAMETERS   10.  -  10.4 ,   ZONAL CURVATURES ARE
 8.8  9.05  9.3  9.6  9.9  10.2  10.5  10.8  11.15  11.5  11.85  12.2  12.55  12.95  13.35  13.75  14.15  14.55  15

FOR EDGE LIFT   0.07 ,   OPTIC DIAMETERS   10.2  -  10.6 ,   ZONAL CURVATURES ARE
 8.6  8.85  9.1  9.4  9.65  9.95  10.25  10.55  10.85  11.2  11.55  11.85  12.2  12.6  12.95  13.35  13.75  14.15  14.55

FOR EDGE LIFT   0.07 ,   OPTIC DIAMETERS   10.4  -  10.8 ,   ZONAL CURVATURES ARE
 8.4  8.65  8.95  9.2  9.45  9.75  10  10.3  10.6  10.9  11.25  11.55  11.9  12.25  12.6  12.95  13.35  13.75  14.15

FOR EDGE LIFT   0.07 ,   OPTIC DIAMETERS   10.6  -  11. ,   ZONAL CURVATURES ARE
 8.25  8.5  8.75  9  9.25  9.55  9.8  10.1  10.35  10.65  11  11.3  11.6  11.95  12.3  12.65  13  13.35  13.75
```

```
FOR EDGE LIFT   0.08 ,   OPTIC DIAMETERS   7 - 7.4 ,   ZONAL CURVATURES ARE
 18.4  19.45  20.6  21.85  23.2  24.7  26.35  28.15  30.15  32.35  34.8  37.6  40.75  44.35  48.55  53.4  59.15  66.05  74.5

FOR EDGE LIFT   0.08 ,   OPTIC DIAMETERS   7.2 - 7.6 ,   ZONAL CURVATURES ARE
 17  17.95  18.95  20  21.2  22.45  23.8  25.25  26.9  28.65  30.6  32.8  35.2  37.9  40.95  44.45  48.4  53.05  58.45

FOR EDGE LIFT   0.08 ,   OPTIC DIAMETERS   7.4 - 7.8 ,   ZONAL CURVATURES ARE
 15.9  16.7  17.55  18.5  19.5  20.6  21.75  23  24.35  25.85  27.45  29.2  31.1  33.25  35.6  38.25  41.2  44.55  48.35

FOR EDGE LIFT   0.08 ,   OPTIC DIAMETERS   7.6 - 8. ,   ZONAL CURVATURES ARE
 14.9  15.65  16.4  17.25  18.15  19.05  20.1  21.15  22.3  23.55  24.95  26.4  28  29.7  31.6  33.7  36.05  38.6  41.5

FOR EDGE LIFT   0.08 ,   OPTIC DIAMETERS   7.8 - 8.2 ,   ZONAL CURVATURES ARE
 14.05  14.75  15.45  16.2  16.95  17.8  18.7  19.65  20.65  21.75  22.9  24.15  25.5  26.95  28.55  30.25  32.15  34.2  36.45

FOR EDGE LIFT   0.08 ,   OPTIC DIAMETERS   8. - 8.4 ,   ZONAL CURVATURES ARE
 13.35  13.95  14.6  15.25  15.95  16.7  17.5  18.35  19.25  20.2  21.2  22.3  23.45  24.7  26.05  27.5  29.1  30.8  32.65

FOR EDGE LIFT   0.08 ,   OPTIC DIAMETERS   8.2 - 8.6 ,   ZONAL CURVATURES ARE
 12.7  13.25  13.85  14.45  15.1  15.8  16.5  17.25  18.05  18.9  19.8  20.75  21.8  22.9  24.05  25.3  26.65  28.05  29.65

FOR EDGE LIFT   0.08 ,   OPTIC DIAMETERS   8.4 - 8.8 ,   ZONAL CURVATURES ARE
 12.15  12.65  13.2  13.75  14.35  14.95  15.6  16.3  17.05  17.8  18.6  19.45  20.35  21.35  22.35  23.45  24.6  25.85  27.2

FOR EDGE LIFT   0.08 ,   OPTIC DIAMETERS   8.6 - 9 ,   ZONAL CURVATURES ARE
 11.65  12.1  12.6  13.15  13.7  14.25  14.85  15.5  16.15  16.85  17.55  18.35  19.15  20  20.95  21.9  22.95  24  25.2
```

```
FOR EDGE LIFT   0.08 ,   OPTIC DIAMETERS   8.8  -  9.2 ,    ZONAL CURVATURES ARE
 11.2  11.65  12.1  12.6  13.1  13.6  14.15  14.75  15.35  16  16.65  17.35  18.1  18.9  19.7  20.6  21.5  22.45  23.5

FOR EDGE LIFT   0.08 ,   OPTIC DIAMETERS   9.  -  9.4 ,    ZONAL CURVATURES ARE
 10.8  11.2  11.65  12.1  12.55  13.05  13.55  14.1  14.65  15.25  15.85  16.5  17.2  17.9  18.65  19.45  20.25  21.15  22.05

FOR EDGE LIFT   0.08 ,   OPTIC DIAMETERS   9.2  -  9.6 ,    ZONAL CURVATURES ARE
 10.4  10.8  11.2  11.65  12.1  12.55  13  13.5  14.05  14.6  15.15  15.75  16.4  17.05  17.7  18.45  19.2  20  20.8

FOR EDGE LIFT   0.08 ,   OPTIC DIAMETERS   9.4  -  9.8 ,    ZONAL CURVATURES ARE
 10.05  10.45  10.85  11.25  11.65  12.1  12.55  13  13.5  14  14.55  15.1  15.65  16.25  16.9  17.55  18.25  18.95  19.75

FOR EDGE LIFT   0.08 ,   OPTIC DIAMETERS   9.6  -  10. ,    ZONAL CURVATURES ARE
 9.75  10.1  10.5  10.85  11.25  11.65  12.1  12.5  13  13.45  13.95  14.45  15  15.55  16.15  16.75  17.4  18.05  18.75

FOR EDGE LIFT   0.08 ,   OPTIC DIAMETERS   9.8  -  10.2 ,    ZONAL CURVATURES ARE
 9.5  9.8  10.15  10.5  10.9  11.3  11.7  12.1  12.55  12.95  13.45  13.9  14.45  14.95  15.5  16.05  16.65  17.3  17.9

FOR EDGE LIFT   0.08 ,   OPTIC DIAMETERS   10.  -  10.4 ,    ZONAL CURVATURES ARE
 9.2  9.55  9.85  10.2  10.55  10.95  11.3  11.7  12.1  12.55  12.95  13.45  13.9  14.4  14.9  15.45  16  16.55  17.15

FOR EDGE LIFT   0.08 ,   OPTIC DIAMETERS   10.2  -  10.6 ,    ZONAL CURVATURES ARE
 9  9.3  9.6  9.9  10.25  10.6  10.95  11.35  11.75  12.15  12.55  12.95  13.4  13.9  14.35  14.85  15.4  15.9  16.5

FOR EDGE LIFT   0.08 ,   OPTIC DIAMETERS   10.4  -  10.8 ,    ZONAL CURVATURES ARE
 8.75  9.05  9.35  9.65  10  10.3  10.65  11  11.4  11.75  12.15  12.55  13  13.4  13.85  14.35  14.85  15.35  15.85

FOR EDGE LIFT   0.08 ,   OPTIC DIAMETERS   10.6  -  11. ,    ZONAL CURVATURES ARE
 8.55  8.85  9.1  9.4  9.75  10.05  10.35  10.7  11.05  11.4  11.8  12.2  12.6  13  13.4  13.85  14.35  14.8  15.3
```

```
FOR EDGE LIFT   0.09 ,   OPTIC DIAMETERS   7 - 7.4 ,   ZONAL CURVATURES ARE
 24.3  26.25  28.5  31  33.85  37.2  41.1  45.75  51.3  58.15  66.8 NE  NE  NE  NE  NE  NE  NE  NE

FOR EDGE LIFT   0.09 ,   OPTIC DIAMETERS   7.2 - 7.6 ,   ZONAL CURVATURES ARE
 21.75  23.3  25.1  27.05  29.25  31.8  34.65  37.95  41.8  46.3  51.75  58.35  66.55 NE  NE  NE  NE  NE  NE

FOR EDGE LIFT   0.09 ,   OPTIC DIAMETERS   7.4 - 7.8 ,   ZONAL CURVATURES ARE
 19.7  21.05  22.5  24.1  25.85  27.85  30.05  32.55  35.4  38.7  42.45  46.9  52.2  58.55  66.4 NE  NE  NE  NE

FOR EDGE LIFT   0.09 ,   OPTIC DIAMETERS   7.6 - 8. ,   ZONAL CURVATURES ARE
 18.05  19.2  20.45  21.75  23.25  24.85  26.65  28.65  30.85  33.35  36.2  39.4  43.15  47.5  52.65  58.85  66.35 NE  NE

FOR EDGE LIFT   0.09 ,   OPTIC DIAMETERS   7.8 - 8.2 ,   ZONAL CURVATURES ARE
 16.7  17.7  18.75  19.9  21.15  22.5  24  25.6  27.4  29.4  31.65  34.15  36.95  40.15  43.85  48.15  53.15  59.15  66.4

FOR EDGE LIFT   0.09 ,   OPTIC DIAMETERS   8. - 8.4 ,   ZONAL CURVATURES ARE
 15.6  16.45  17.35  18.35  19.45  20.6  21.85  23.25  24.75  26.4  28.2  30.2  32.45  34.95  37.75  40.9  44.55  48.75  53.7

FOR EDGE LIFT   0.09 ,   OPTIC DIAMETERS   8.2 - 8.6 ,   ZONAL CURVATURES ARE
 14.6  15.4  16.2  17.1  18.05  19.05  20.15  21.3  22.6  24  25.5  27.15  29  31  33.25  35.7  38.5  41.65  45.25

FOR EDGE LIFT   0.09 ,   OPTIC DIAMETERS   8.4 - 8.8 ,   ZONAL CURVATURES ARE
 13.75  14.45  15.2  16  16.85  17.75  18.7  19.75  20.85  22.05  23.35  24.75  26.25  27.95  29.75  31.8  34  36.5  39.3

FOR EDGE LIFT   0.09 ,   OPTIC DIAMETERS   8.6 - 9 ,   ZONAL CURVATURES ARE
 13.05  13.7  14.35  15.05  15.8  16.6  17.45  18.4  19.35  20.4  21.55  22.75  24.05  25.5  27.05  28.7  30.55  32.6  34.8
```

```
FOR EDGE LIFT   0.09 ,   OPTIC DIAMETERS   8.8  -  9.2 ,    ZONAL CURVATURES ARE
 12.4  13  13.6  14.25  14.95  15.65  16.4  17.25  18.1  19.05  20.05  21.1  22.25  23.45  24.8  26.25  27.8  29.5  31.35

FOR EDGE LIFT   0.09 ,   OPTIC DIAMETERS   9.  -  9.4 ,    ZONAL CURVATURES ARE
 11.85  12.35  12.95  13.5  14.15  14.8  15.5  16.25  17.05  17.85  18.75  19.7  20.7  21.8  22.95  24.2  25.55  27  28.55

FOR EDGE LIFT   0.09 ,   OPTIC DIAMETERS   9.2  -  9.6 ,    ZONAL CURVATURES ARE
 11.3  11.8  12.35  12.9  13.45  14.05  14.7  15.4  16.1  16.85  17.65  18.5  19.4  20.35  21.4  22.5  23.65  24.9  26.25

FOR EDGE LIFT   0.09 ,   OPTIC DIAMETERS   9.4  -  9.8 ,    ZONAL CURVATURES ARE
 10.85  11.35  11.8  12.3  12.85  13.4  14  14.65  15.3  15.95  16.7  17.45  18.3  19.15  20.05  21.05  22.1  23.2  24.35

FOR EDGE LIFT   0.09 ,   OPTIC DIAMETERS   9.6  -  10. ,    ZONAL CURVATURES ARE
 10.45  10.9  11.35  11.8  12.3  12.85  13.4  13.95  14.55  15.2  15.85  16.55  17.3  18.1  18.9  19.8  20.7  21.7  22.75

FOR EDGE LIFT   0.09 ,   OPTIC DIAMETERS   9.8  -  10.2 ,    ZONAL CURVATURES ARE
 10.1  10.5  10.9  11.35  11.8  12.3  12.8  13.35  13.9  14.5  15.1  15.75  16.45  17.15  17.9  18.7  19.55  20.45  21.4

FOR EDGE LIFT   0.09 ,   OPTIC DIAMETERS   10.  -  10.4 ,    ZONAL CURVATURES ARE
 9.75  10.15  10.55  10.95  11.4  11.85  12.3  12.8  13.3  13.85  14.45  15.05  15.65  16.3  17  17.75  18.5  19.3  20.2

FOR EDGE LIFT   0.09 ,   OPTIC DIAMETERS   10.2  -  10.6 ,    ZONAL CURVATURES ARE
 9.45  9.8  10.15  10.55  11  11.4  11.85  12.3  12.8  13.3  13.85  14.4  14.95  15.6  16.2  16.9  17.6  18.35  19.1

FOR EDGE LIFT   0.09 ,   OPTIC DIAMETERS   10.4  -  10.8 ,    ZONAL CURVATURES ARE
 9.15  9.5  9.85  10.2  10.6  11  11.45  11.85  12.3  12.8  13.3  13.8  14.35  14.9  15.5  16.15  16.8  17.45  18.2

FOR EDGE LIFT   0.09 ,   OPTIC DIAMETERS   10.6  -  11. ,    ZONAL CURVATURES ARE
 8.9  9.25  9.55  9.9  10.3  10.65  11.05  11.45  11.9  12.35  12.8  13.3  13.8  14.35  14.9  15.45  16.05  16.7  17.35
```

```
FOR EDGE LIFT   0.1 ,   OPTIC DIAMETERS   7  -  7.4 ,    ZONAL CURVATURES ARE
 36.25  40.9  46.6  53.9  63.35 NE  NE  NE  NE  NE  NE  NE  NE  NE  NE  NE  NE  NE  NE

FOR EDGE LIFT   0.1 ,   OPTIC DIAMETERS   7.2  -  7.6 ,    ZONAL CURVATURES ARE
 30.35  33.65  37.5  42.15  47.9  55.15 NE  NE  NE  NE  NE  NE  NE  NE  NE  NE  NE  NE  NE

FOR EDGE LIFT   0.1 ,   OPTIC DIAMETERS   7.4  -  7.8 ,    ZONAL CURVATURES ARE
 26.2  28.65  31.5  34.85  38.75  43.45  49.2  56.4 NE  NE  NE  NE  NE  NE  NE  NE  NE  NE  NE

FOR EDGE LIFT   0.1 ,   OPTIC DIAMETERS   7.6  -  8. ,    ZONAL CURVATURES ARE
 23.15  25.05  27.25  29.8  32.65  36.05  40  44.75  50.5  57.7 NE  NE  NE  NE  NE  NE  NE  NE  NE

FOR EDGE LIFT   0.1 ,   OPTIC DIAMETERS   7.8  -  8.2 ,    ZONAL CURVATURES ARE
 20.75  22.35  24.1  26.1  28.35  30.9  33.85  37.25  41.25  46  51.8  59 NE  NE  NE  NE  NE  NE  NE

FOR EDGE LIFT   0.1 ,   OPTIC DIAMETERS   8.  -  8.4 ,    ZONAL CURVATURES ARE
 18.85  20.2  21.65  23.25  25.1  27.1  29.4  32  35  38.45  42.5  47.3  53.1  60.25 NE  NE  NE  NE  NE

FOR EDGE LIFT   0.1 ,   OPTIC DIAMETERS   8.2  -  8.6 ,    ZONAL CURVATURES ARE
 17.3  18.45  19.7  21.05  22.55  24.2  26.1  28.15  30.5  33.15  36.15  39.65  43.75  48.6  54.4  61.55 NE  NE  NE

FOR EDGE LIFT   0.1 ,   OPTIC DIAMETERS   8.4  -  8.8 ,    ZONAL CURVATURES ARE
 16  17  18.1  19.25  20.55  21.95  23.5  25.2  27.05  29.2  31.55  34.25  37.35  40.9  45  49.9  55.7  62.8 NE

FOR EDGE LIFT   0.1 ,   OPTIC DIAMETERS   8.6  -  9 ,    ZONAL CURVATURES ARE
 14.95  15.8  16.75  17.75  18.9  20.1  21.4  22.85  24.4  26.15  28.1  30.25  32.65  35.4  38.5  42.1  46.25  51.15  57
```

FOR EDGE LIFT 0.1 , OPTIC DIAMETERS 8.8 - 9.2 , ZONAL CURVATURES ARE

14 14.8 15.6 16.5 17.5 18.55 19.7 20.9 22.25 23.75 25.35 27.1 29.1 31.3 33.75 36.55 39.7 43.3 47.5

FOR EDGE LIFT 0.1 , OPTIC DIAMETERS 9. - 9.4 , ZONAL CURVATURES ARE

13.2 13.9 14.65 15.45 16.3 17.25 18.25 19.3 20.5 21.75 23.15 24.65 26.3 28.1 30.1 32.35 34.85 37.7 40.9

FOR EDGE LIFT 0.1 , OPTIC DIAMETERS 9.2 - 9.6 , ZONAL CURVATURES ARE

12.5 13.15 13.8 14.55 15.3 16.15 17.05 18 19 20.1 21.3 22.6 24 25.55 27.25 29.1 31.15 33.4 35.95

FOR EDGE LIFT 0.1 , OPTIC DIAMETERS 9.4 - 9.8 , ZONAL CURVATURES ARE

11.85 12.45 13.05 13.75 14.45 15.2 16 16.85 17.75 18.75 19.8 20.9 22.15 23.45 24.9 26.5 28.2 30.1 32.15

FOR EDGE LIFT 0.1 , OPTIC DIAMETERS 9.6 - 10. , ZONAL CURVATURES ARE

11.3 11.85 12.45 13.05 13.65 14.35 15.1 15.85 16.65 17.55 18.5 19.5 20.55 21.7 22.95 24.35 25.8 27.4 29.15

FOR EDGE LIFT 0.1 , OPTIC DIAMETERS 9.8 - 10.2 , ZONAL CURVATURES ARE

10.8 11.3 11.85 12.4 13 13.6 14.3 15 15.7 16.5 17.35 18.25 19.2 20.25 21.35 22.55 23.8 25.2 26.7

FOR EDGE LIFT 0.1 , OPTIC DIAMETERS 10. - 10.4 , ZONAL CURVATURES ARE

10.4 10.85 11.35 11.85 12.4 12.95 13.6 14.2 14.9 15.6 16.4 17.2 18.05 19 19.95 21 22.15 23.35 24.65

FOR EDGE LIFT 0.1 , OPTIC DIAMETERS 10.2 - 10.6 , ZONAL CURVATURES ARE

10 10.4 10.85 11.35 11.85 12.4 12.95 13.55 14.15 14.8 15.5 16.25 17.05 17.9 18.75 19.7 20.7 21.8 22.95

FOR EDGE LIFT 0.1 , OPTIC DIAMETERS 10.4 - 10.8 , ZONAL CURVATURES ARE

9.65 10.05 10.45 10.9 11.35 11.85 12.4 12.95 13.5 14.1 14.75 15.45 16.15 16.9 17.7 18.6 19.5 20.45 21.5

FOR EDGE LIFT 0.1 , OPTIC DIAMETERS 10.6 - 11. , ZONAL CURVATURES ARE

9.3 9.7 10.1 10.5 10.95 11.4 11.9 12.4 12.95 13.5 14.1 14.7 15.35 16.05 16.8 17.6 18.4 19.3 20.2

```
FOR EDGE LIFT   0.11 ,   OPTIC DIAMETERS   7  -  7.4 ,    ZONAL CURVATURES ARE
NE  NE  NE  NE  NE  NE  NE  NE  NE  NE  NE  NE  NE  NE  NE  NE  NE  NE  NE

FOR EDGE LIFT   0.11 ,   OPTIC DIAMETERS   7.2  -  7.6 ,    ZONAL CURVATURES ARE
 50.95  61.05 NE  NE  NE  NE  NE  NE  NE  NE  NE  NE  NE  NE  NE  NE  NE  NE  NE

FOR EDGE LIFT   0.11 ,   OPTIC DIAMETERS   7.4  -  7.8 ,    ZONAL CURVATURES ARE
 39.55  45.55  53.3  63.7 NE  NE  NE  NE  NE  NE  NE  NE  NE  NE  NE  NE  NE  NE  NE

FOR EDGE LIFT   0.11 ,   OPTIC DIAMETERS   7.6  -  8. ,    ZONAL CURVATURES ARE
 32.45  36.5  41.45  47.65  55.65 NE  NE  NE  NE  NE  NE  NE  NE  NE  NE  NE  NE  NE  NE

FOR EDGE LIFT   0.11 ,   OPTIC DIAMETERS   7.8  -  8.2 ,    ZONAL CURVATURES ARE
 27.6  30.55  34.05  38.25  43.4  49.8  58.05 NE  NE  NE  NE  NE  NE  NE  NE  NE  NE  NE  NE

FOR EDGE LIFT   0.11 ,   OPTIC DIAMETERS   8.  -  8.4 ,    ZONAL CURVATURES ARE
 24.1  26.35  29  32.05  35.7  40.05  45.35  51.95  60.45 NE  NE  NE  NE  NE  NE  NE  NE  NE  NE

FOR EDGE LIFT   0.11 ,   OPTIC DIAMETERS   8.2  -  8.6 ,    ZONAL CURVATURES ARE
 21.4  23.25  25.3  27.65  30.4  33.6  37.35  41.85  47.3  54.15  62.9 NE  NE  NE  NE  NE  NE  NE  NE

FOR EDGE LIFT   0.11 ,   OPTIC DIAMETERS   8.4  -  8.8 ,    ZONAL CURVATURES ARE
 19.3  20.8  22.5  24.4  26.55  29  31.85  35.15  39  43.65  49.35  56.35 NE  NE  NE  NE  NE  NE  NE

FOR EDGE LIFT   0.11 ,   OPTIC DIAMETERS   8.6  -  9 ,    ZONAL CURVATURES ARE
 17.6  18.85  20.3  21.85  23.6  25.6  27.8  30.35  33.3  36.7  40.75  45.55  51.35  58.6 NE  NE  NE  NE  NE
```

FOR EDGE LIFT 0.11 , OPTIC DIAMETERS 8.8 - 9.2 , ZONAL CURVATURES ARE

16.2 17.3 18.5 19.85 21.3 22.95 24.75 26.8 29.1 31.75 34.8 38.3 42.45 47.4 53.45 60.9 NE NE NE

FOR EDGE LIFT 0.11 , OPTIC DIAMETERS 9. - 9.4 , ZONAL CURVATURES ARE

15 15.95 17 18.15 19.4 20.8 22.35 24 25.9 28.05 30.45 33.15 36.3 39.95 44.25 49.35 55.5 63.15 NE

FOR EDGE LIFT 0.11 , OPTIC DIAMETERS 9.2 - 9.6 , ZONAL CURVATURES ARE

14 14.85 15.8 16.8 17.9 19.05 20.35 21.8 23.4 25.15 27.1 29.3 31.75 34.6 37.85 41.6 46 51.25 57.65

FOR EDGE LIFT 0.11 , OPTIC DIAMETERS 9.4 - 9.8 , ZONAL CURVATURES ARE

13.15 13.9 14.75 15.6 16.6 17.6 18.75 20 21.35 22.8 24.45 26.25 28.3 30.55 33.15 36.05 39.4 43.25 47.85

FOR EDGE LIFT 0.11 , OPTIC DIAMETERS 9.6 - 10. , ZONAL CURVATURES ARE

12.4 13.1 13.8 14.6 15.45 16.4 17.4 18.45 19.65 20.9 22.3 23.85 25.55 27.45 29.5 31.85 34.5 37.55 41

FOR EDGE LIFT 0.11 , OPTIC DIAMETERS 9.8 - 10.2 , ZONAL CURVATURES ARE

11.75 12.35 13.05 13.75 14.5 15.35 16.25 17.2 18.2 19.35 20.55 21.9 23.3 24.9 26.65 28.6 30.75 33.2 35.9

FOR EDGE LIFT 0.11 , OPTIC DIAMETERS 10. - 10.4 , ZONAL CURVATURES ARE

11.15 11.75 12.35 13 13.7 14.45 15.25 16.1 17 18 19.05 20.2 21.5 22.85 24.35 26 27.8 29.8 32.05

FOR EDGE LIFT 0.11 , OPTIC DIAMETERS 10.2 - 10.6 , ZONAL CURVATURES ARE

10.65 11.15 11.75 12.35 12.95 13.65 14.35 15.15 15.95 16.85 17.8 18.8 19.95 21.1 22.4 23.85 25.4 27.1 28.95

FOR EDGE LIFT 0.11 , OPTIC DIAMETERS 10.4 - 10.8 , ZONAL CURVATURES ARE

10.2 10.65 11.2 11.75 12.3 12.95 13.6 14.3 15.05 15.85 16.7 17.6 18.6 19.65 20.8 22.05 23.4 24.85 26.45

FOR EDGE LIFT 0.11 , OPTIC DIAMETERS 10.6 - 11. , ZONAL CURVATURES ARE

9.75 10.2 10.7 11.2 11.75 12.3 12.9 13.55 14.25 14.95 15.75 16.55 17.45 18.4 19.4 20.5 21.7 23 24.35

```
FOR EDGE LIFT   0.12 ,   OPTIC DIAMETERS   7 - 7.4 ,   ZONAL CURVATURES ARE
NE  NE  NE  NE  NE  NE  NE  NE  NE  NE  NE  NE  NE  NE  NE  NE  NE  NE  NE

FOR EDGE LIFT   0.12 ,   OPTIC DIAMETERS   7.2 - 7.6 ,   ZONAL CURVATURES ARE
NE  NE  NE  NE  NE  NE  NE  NE  NE  NE  NE  NE  NE  NE  NE  NE  NE  NE  NE

FOR EDGE LIFT   0.12 ,   OPTIC DIAMETERS   7.4 - 7.8 ,   ZONAL CURVATURES ARE
 81.75 NE  NE  NE  NE  NE  NE  NE  NE  NE  NE  NE  NE  NE  NE  NE  NE  NE  NE

FOR EDGE LIFT   0.12 ,   OPTIC DIAMETERS   7.6 - 8. ,   ZONAL CURVATURES ARE
 55  67.95 NE  NE  NE  NE  NE  NE  NE  NE  NE  NE  NE  NE  NE  NE  NE  NE  NE

FOR EDGE LIFT   0.12 ,   OPTIC DIAMETERS   7.8 - 8.2 ,   ZONAL CURVATURES ARE
 41.65  48.9  58.7  72.6 NE  NE  NE  NE  NE  NE  NE  NE  NE  NE  NE  NE  NE  NE  NE

FOR EDGE LIFT   0.12 ,   OPTIC DIAMETERS   8. - 8.4 ,   ZONAL CURVATURES ARE
 33.65  38.35  44.35  52.1  62.55  77.5 NE  NE  NE  NE  NE  NE  NE  NE  NE  NE  NE  NE  NE

FOR EDGE LIFT   0.12 ,   OPTIC DIAMETERS   8.2 - 8.6 ,   ZONAL CURVATURES ARE
 28.3  31.65  35.75  40.75  47.1  55.4  66.6  82.6 NE  NE  NE  NE  NE  NE  NE  NE  NE  NE  NE

FOR EDGE LIFT   0.12 ,   OPTIC DIAMETERS   8.4 - 8.8 ,   ZONAL CURVATURES ARE
 24.45  27  30  33.6  37.9  43.25  50  58.8  70.75 NE  NE  NE  NE  NE  NE  NE  NE  NE  NE

FOR EDGE LIFT   0.12 ,   OPTIC DIAMETERS   8.6 - 9 ,   ZONAL CURVATURES ARE
 21.55  23.6  25.9  28.65  31.8  35.6  40.15  45.85  53  62.4  75.15 NE  NE  NE  NE  NE  NE  NE  NE
```

```
FOR EDGE LIFT   0.12 ,   OPTIC DIAMETERS   8.8  -  9.2 ,    ZONAL CURVATURES ARE
 19.3  21  22.85  25  27.45  30.3  33.65  37.65  42.5  48.5  56.1  66.1  79.7 NE  NE  NE  NE  NE  NE

FOR EDGE LIFT   0.12 ,   OPTIC DIAMETERS   9.  -  9.4 ,    ZONAL CURVATURES ARE
 17.5  18.9  20.45  22.2  24.2  26.45  29  32.05  35.6  39.8  44.95  51.3  59.35  69.95  84.4 NE  NE  NE  NE

FOR EDGE LIFT   0.12 ,   OPTIC DIAMETERS   9.2  -  9.6 ,    ZONAL CURVATURES ARE
 16.05  17.25  18.55  20  21.65  23.5  25.55  27.9  30.65  33.8  37.55  42  47.45  54.15  62.7  73.9  89.35 NE  NE

FOR EDGE LIFT   0.12 ,   OPTIC DIAMETERS   9.4  -  9.8 ,    ZONAL CURVATURES ARE
 14.8  15.85  17  18.25  19.6  21.15  22.85  24.8  26.95  29.45  32.35  35.65  39.6  44.3  50  57.1  66.15  78.05 NE

FOR EDGE LIFT   0.12 ,   OPTIC DIAMETERS   9.6  -  10. ,    ZONAL CURVATURES ARE
 13.8  14.7  15.65  16.75  17.95  19.25  20.7  22.3  24.1  26.15  28.4  31.05  34.05  37.55  41.7  46.65  52.7  60.15  69.75

FOR EDGE LIFT   0.12 ,   OPTIC DIAMETERS   9.8  -  10.2 ,    ZONAL CURVATURES ARE
 12.9  13.7  14.55  15.5  16.55  17.7  18.95  20.3  21.8  23.5  25.4  27.5  29.95  32.65  35.85  39.55  43.9  49.1  55.45

FOR EDGE LIFT   0.12 ,   OPTIC DIAMETERS   10.  -  10.4 ,    ZONAL CURVATURES ARE
 12.1  12.85  13.6  14.45  15.4  16.4  17.45  18.65  19.95  21.4  23  24.75  26.7  28.95  31.45  34.35  37.7  41.55  46.1

FOR EDGE LIFT   0.12 ,   OPTIC DIAMETERS   10.2  -  10.6 ,    ZONAL CURVATURES ARE
 11.45  12.1  12.8  13.55  14.4  15.25  16.2  17.25  18.4  19.65  21  22.5  24.15  26  28.1  30.4  33.05  36.1  39.55

FOR EDGE LIFT   0.12 ,   OPTIC DIAMETERS   10.4  -  10.8 ,    ZONAL CURVATURES ARE
 10.85  11.45  12.1  12.75  13.5  14.3  15.15  16.1  17.1  18.15  19.35  20.65  22.1  23.65  25.4  27.35  29.5  31.95  34.7

FOR EDGE LIFT   0.12 ,   OPTIC DIAMETERS   10.6  -  11. ,    ZONAL CURVATURES ARE
 10.35  10.9  11.45  12.1  12.75  13.45  14.25  15.05  15.95  16.9  17.95  19.1  20.35  21.7  23.2  24.85  26.65  28.65  30.95
```

```
FOR EDGE LIFT   0.13 ,   OPTIC DIAMETERS   7  -  7.4 ,    ZONAL CURVATURES ARE
NE  NE  NE  NE  NE  NE  NE  NE  NE  NE  NE  NE  NE  NE  NE  NE  NE  NE  NE

FOR EDGE LIFT   0.13 ,   OPTIC DIAMETERS   7.2  -  7.6 ,    ZONAL CURVATURES ARE
NE  NE  NE  NE  NE  NE  NE  NE  NE  NE  NE  NE  NE  NE  NE  NE  NE  NE  NE

FOR EDGE LIFT   0.13 ,   OPTIC DIAMETERS   7.4  -  7.8 ,    ZONAL CURVATURES ARE
NE  NE  NE  NE  NE  NE  NE  NE  NE  NE  NE  NE  NE  NE  NE  NE  NE  NE  NE

FOR EDGE LIFT   0.13 ,   OPTIC DIAMETERS   7.6  -  8. ,    ZONAL CURVATURES ARE
NE  NE  NE  NE  NE  NE  NE  NE  NE  NE  NE  NE  NE  NE  NE  NE  NE  NE  NE

FOR EDGE LIFT   0.13 ,   OPTIC DIAMETERS   7.8  -  8.2 ,    ZONAL CURVATURES ARE
NE  NE  NE  NE  NE  NE  NE  NE  NE  NE  NE  NE  NE  NE  NE  NE  NE  NE  NE

FOR EDGE LIFT   0.13 ,   OPTIC DIAMETERS   8.  -  8.4 ,    ZONAL CURVATURES ARE
 56.45  71.45 NE  NE  NE  NE  NE  NE  NE  NE  NE  NE  NE  NE  NE  NE  NE  NE  NE

FOR EDGE LIFT   0.13 ,   OPTIC DIAMETERS   8.2  -  8.6 ,    ZONAL CURVATURES ARE
 42.15  50.25  61.6  78.5 NE  NE  NE  NE  NE  NE  NE  NE  NE  NE  NE  NE  NE  NE  NE

FOR EDGE LIFT   0.13 ,   OPTIC DIAMETERS   8.4  -  8.8 ,    ZONAL CURVATURES ARE
 33.7  38.9  45.6  54.55  67.15  86.3 NE  NE  NE  NE  NE  NE  NE  NE  NE  NE  NE  NE  NE

FOR EDGE LIFT   0.13 ,   OPTIC DIAMETERS   8.6  -  9 ,    ZONAL CURVATURES ARE
 28.1  31.75  36.25  41.9  49.25  59.15  73.25 NE  NE  NE  NE  NE  NE  NE  NE  NE  NE  NE  NE
```

```
FOR EDGE LIFT   0.13 ,   OPTIC DIAMETERS   8.8  -  9.2 ,    ZONAL CURVATURES ARE
 24.15  26.9  30.15  34.1  39  45.15  53.2  64.15  79.85 NE  NE  NE  NE  NE  NE  NE  NE  NE  NE

FOR EDGE LIFT   0.13 ,   OPTIC DIAMETERS   9.  -  9.4 ,    ZONAL CURVATURES ARE
 21.2  23.35  25.85  28.8  32.35  36.6  41.9  43.6  57.4  69.5  87.05 NE  NE  NE  NE  NE  NE  NE  NE

FOR EDGE LIFT   0.13 ,   OPTIC DIAMETERS   9.2  -  9.6 ,    ZONAL CURVATURES ARE
 18.95  20.65  22.65  24.95  27.65  30.8  34.6  39.2  44.95  52.25  61.9  75.25 NE  NE  NE  NE  NE  NE  NE

FOR EDGE LIFT   0.13 ,   OPTIC DIAMETERS   9.4  -  9.8 ,    ZONAL CURVATURES ARE
 17.1  18.55  20.2  22.05  24.2  26.65  29.5  32.9  37  41.95  48.15  56.15  66.75  81.5 NE  NE  NE  NE  NE

FOR EDGE LIFT   0.13 ,   OPTIC DIAMETERS   9.6  -  10. ,    ZONAL CURVATURES ARE
 15.6  16.85  18.2  19.75  21.5  23.5  25.75  28.4  31.5  35.1  39.5  44.85  51.6  60.3  71.9  88.25 NE  NE  NE

FOR EDGE LIFT   0.13 ,   OPTIC DIAMETERS   9.8  -  10.2 ,    ZONAL CURVATURES ARE
 14.35  15.45  16.6  17.95  19.4  21.05  22.9  25  27.45  30.25  33.55  37.45  42.15  47.95  55.25  64.7  77.45 NE  NE

FOR EDGE LIFT   0.13 ,   OPTIC DIAMETERS   10.  -  10.4 ,    ZONAL CURVATURES ARE
 13.35  14.25  15.3  16.4  17.65  19.05  20.6  22.35  24.35  26.6  29.15  32.15  35.7  39.85  44.95  51.2  59.1  69.4  83.4

FOR EDGE LIFT   0.13 ,   OPTIC DIAMETERS   10.2  -  10.6 ,    ZONAL CURVATURES ARE
 12.45  13.25  14.15  15.15  16.25  17.45  18.75  20.25  21.9  23.75  25.85  28.2  30.95  34.15  37.95  42.4  47.85  54.6
 63.2

FOR EDGE LIFT   0.13 ,   OPTIC DIAMETERS   10.4  -  10.8 ,    ZONAL CURVATURES ARE
 11.65  12.4  13.2  14.1  15.05  16.1  17.25  18.5  19.9  21.45  23.2  25.15  27.4  29.95  32.85  36.25  40.3  45.1  50.95

FOR EDGE LIFT   0.13 ,   OPTIC DIAMETERS   10.6  -  11. ,    ZONAL CURVATURES ARE
 11  11.65  12.4  13.15  14  14.95  15.95  17.05  18.25  19.6  21.05  22.7  24.55  26.65  29  31.7  34.85  38.45  42.75
```

FOR EDGE LIFT 0.14 , OPTIC DIAMETERS 7 - 7.4 , ZONAL CURVATURES ARE

NE NE NE NE NE NE NE NE NE NE NE NE NE NE NE NE NE NE NE

FOR EDGE LIFT 0.14 , OPTIC DIAMETERS 7.2 - 7.6 , ZONAL CURVATURES ARE

NE NE NE NE NE NE NE NE NE NE NE NE NE NE NE NE NE NE NE

FOR EDGE LIFT 0.14 , OPTIC DIAMETERS 7.4 - 7.8 , ZONAL CURVATURES ARE

NE NE NE NE NE NE NE NE NE NE NE NE NE NE NE NE NE NE NE

FOR EDGE LIFT 0.14 , OPTIC DIAMETERS 7.6 - 8. , ZONAL CURVATURES ARE

NE NE NE NE NE NE NE NE NE NE NE NE NE NE NE NE NE NE NE

FOR EDGE LIFT 0.14 , OPTIC DIAMETERS 7.8 - 8.2 , ZONAL CURVATURES ARE

NE NE NE NE NE NE NE NE NE NE NE NE NE NE NE NE NE NE NE

FOR EDGE LIFT 0.14 , OPTIC DIAMETERS 8. - 8.4 , ZONAL CURVATURES ARE

NE NE NE NE NE NE NE NE NE NE NE NE NE NE NE NE NE NE NE

FOR EDGE LIFT 0.14 , OPTIC DIAMETERS 8.2 - 8.6 , ZONAL CURVATURES ARE

NE NE NE NE NE NE NE NE NE NE NE NE NE NE NE NE NE NE NE

FOR EDGE LIFT 0.14 , OPTIC DIAMETERS 8.4 - 8.8 , ZONAL CURVATURES ARE

54.8 NE NE NE NE NE NE NE NE NE NE NE NE NE NE NE NE NE NE

FOR EDGE LIFT 0.14 , OPTIC DIAMETERS 8.6 - 9 , ZONAL CURVATURES ARE

40.8 49.2 61.05 NE NE NE NE NE NE NE NE NE NE NE NE NE NE NE NE

```
FOR EDGE LIFT   0.14 ,   OPTIC DIAMETERS   8.8  -  9.2 ,    ZONAL CURVATURES ARE
 32.55  37.9  44.85  54.35 NE  NE  NE  NE  NE  NE  NE  NE  NE  NE  NE  NE  NE  NE  NE

FOR EDGE LIFT   0.14 ,   OPTIC DIAMETERS   9.  -  9.4 ,    ZONAL CURVATURES ARE
 27.1  30.85  35.5  41.4  49.25  60.15 NE  NE  NE  NE  NE  NE  NE  NE  NE  NE  NE  NE  NE

FOR EDGE LIFT   0.14 ,   OPTIC DIAMETERS   9.2  -  9.6 ,    ZONAL CURVATURES ARE
 23.25  26.05  29.4  33.5  38.65  45.3  54.15 NE  NE  NE  NE  NE  NE  NE  NE  NE  NE  NE  NE

FOR EDGE LIFT   0.14 ,   OPTIC DIAMETERS   9.4  -  9.8 ,    ZONAL CURVATURES ARE
 20.35  22.55  25.1  28.15  31.85  36.35  42.1  49.5  59.55 NE  NE  NE  NE  NE  NE  NE  NE  NE  NE

FOR EDGE LIFT   0.14 ,   OPTIC DIAMETERS   9.6  -  10. ,    ZONAL CURVATURES ARE
 18.15  19.9  21.95  24.3  27.1  30.4  34.45  39.45  45.8  54.15 NE  NE  NE  NE  NE  NE  NE  NE  NE

FOR EDGE LIFT   0.14 ,   OPTIC DIAMETERS   9.8  -  10.2 ,    ZONAL CURVATURES ARE
 16.35  17.8  19.5  21.4  23.6  26.15  29.2  32.85  37.25  42.8  49.85  59.2 NE  NE  NE  NE  NE  NE  NE

FOR EDGE LIFT   0.14 ,   OPTIC DIAMETERS   10.  -  10.4 ,    ZONAL CURVATURES ARE
 14.9  16.15  17.55  19.1  20.9  22.95  25.35  28.15  31.45  35.4  40.3  46.4  54.25 NE  NE  NE  NE  NE  NE

FOR EDGE LIFT   0.14 ,   OPTIC DIAMETERS   10.2  -  10.6 ,    ZONAL CURVATURES ARE
 13.7  14.75  15.95  17.3  18.8  20.5  22.4  24.65  27.2  30.25  33.85  38.2  43.55  50.3  59.05 NE  NE  NE  NE

FOR EDGE LIFT   0.14 ,   OPTIC DIAMETERS   10.4  -  10.8 ,    ZONAL CURVATURES ARE
 12.7  13.6  14.65  15.8  17.05  18.5  20.1  21.9  24  26.4  29.2  32.45  36.4  41.15  47  54.5 NE  NE  NE

FOR EDGE LIFT   0.14 ,   OPTIC DIAMETERS   10.6  -  11. ,    ZONAL CURVATURES ARE
 11.85  12.65  13.55  14.55  15.65  16.85  18.25  19.75  21.5  23.45  25.7  28.25  31.3  34.85  39.1  44.3  50.8  59.1 NE
```

```
FOR EDGE LIFT   0.15 ,   OPTIC DIAMETERS   7  -  7.4 ,    ZONAL CURVATURES ARE
NE  NE  NE  NE  NE  NE  NE  NE  NE  NE  NE  NE  NE  NE  NE  NE  NE  NE  NE

FOR EDGE LIFT   0.15 ,   OPTIC DIAMETERS   7.2  -  7.6 ,    ZONAL CURVATURES ARE
NE  NE  NE  NE  NE  NE  NE  NE  NE  NE  NE  NE  NE  NE  NE  NE  NE  NE  NE

FOR EDGE LIFT   0.15 ,   OPTIC DIAMETERS   7.4  -  7.8 ,    ZONAL CURVATURES ARE
NE  NE  NE  NE  NE  NE  NE  NE  NE  NE  NE  NE  NE  NE  NE  NE  NE  NE  NE

FOR EDGE LIFT   0.15 ,   OPTIC DIAMETERS   7.6  -  8. ,    ZONAL CURVATURES ARE
NE  NE  NE  NE  NE  NE  NE  NE  NE  NE  NE  NE  NE  NE  NE  NE  NE  NE  NE

FOR EDGE LIFT   0.15 ,   OPTIC DIAMETERS   7.8  -  8.2 ,    ZONAL CURVATURES ARE
NE  NE  NE  NE  NE  NE  NE  NE  NE  NE  NE  NE  NE  NE  NE  NE  NE  NE  NE

FOR EDGE LIFT   0.15 ,   OPTIC DIAMETERS   8.  -  8.4 ,    ZONAL CURVATURES ARE
NE  NE  NE  NE  NE  NE  NE  NE  NE  NE  NE  NE  NE  NE  NE  NE  NE  NE  NE

FOR EDGE LIFT   0.15 ,   OPTIC DIAMETERS   8.2  -  8.6 ,    ZONAL CURVATURES ARE
NE  NE  NE  NE  NE  NE  NE  NE  NE  NE  NE  NE  NE  NE  NE  NE  NE  NE  NE

FOR EDGE LIFT   0.15 ,   OPTIC DIAMETERS   8.4  -  8.8 ,    ZONAL CURVATURES ARE
NE  NE  NE  NE  NE  NE  NE  NE  NE  NE  NE  NE  NE  NE  NE  NE  NE  NE  NE

FOR EDGE LIFT   0.15 ,   OPTIC DIAMETERS   8.6  -  9 ,    ZONAL CURVATURES ARE
NE  NE  NE  NE  NE  NE  NE  NE  NE  NE  NE  NE  NE  NE  NE  NE  NE  NE  NE
```

FOR EDGE LIFT 0.15 , OPTIC DIAMETERS 8.8 - 9.2 , ZONAL CURVATURES ARE

50.5 NE NE NE NE NE NE NE NE NE NE NE NE NE NE NE NE NE NE

FOR EDGE LIFT 0.15 , OPTIC DIAMETERS 9. - 9.4 , ZONAL CURVATURES ARE

37.95 45.85 57.2 NE NE NE NE NE NE NE NE NE NE NE NE NE NE NE NE

FOR EDGE LIFT 0.15 , OPTIC DIAMETERS 9.2 - 9.6 , ZONAL CURVATURES ARE

30.45 35.55 42.25 51.5 NE NE NE NE NE NE NE NE NE NE NE NE NE NE NE

FOR EDGE LIFT 0.15 , OPTIC DIAMETERS 9.4 - 9.8 , ZONAL CURVATURES ARE

25.4 29 33.5 39.3 47.1 57.95 NE NE NE NE NE NE NE NE NE NE NE NE NE

FOR EDGE LIFT 0.15 , OPTIC DIAMETERS 9.6 - 10. , ZONAL CURVATURES ARE

21.8 24.5 27.8 31.8 36.9 43.55 52.55 NE NE NE NE NE NE NE NE NE NE NE NE

FOR EDGE LIFT 0.15 , OPTIC DIAMETERS 9.8 - 10.2 , ZONAL CURVATURES ARE

19.1 21.25 23.75 26.75 30.4 34.9 40.7 48.3 58.75 NE NE NE NE NE NE NE NE NE NE

FOR EDGE LIFT 0.15 , OPTIC DIAMETERS 10. - 10.4 , ZONAL CURVATURES ARE

17 18.75 20.75 23.05 25.8 29.15 33.2 38.3 44.9 53.65 NE NE NE NE NE NE NE NE NE

FOR EDGE LIFT 0.15 , OPTIC DIAMETERS 10.2 - 10.6 , ZONAL CURVATURES ARE

15.35 16.75 18.4 20.3 22.45 25 28.1 31.75 36.3 42.05 49.55 59.65 NE NE NE NE NE NE NE

FOR EDGE LIFT 0.15 , OPTIC DIAMETERS 10.4 - 10.8 , ZONAL CURVATURES ARE

14 15.2 16.55 18.1 19.9 21.95 24.3 27.15 30.5 34.6 39.7 46.2 54.75 NE NE NE NE NE NE

FOR EDGE LIFT 0.15 , OPTIC DIAMETERS 10.6 - 11. , ZONAL CURVATURES ARE

12.85 13.9 15.05 16.35 17.85 19.5 21.45 23.7 26.3 29.4 33.15 37.7 43.45 50.8 60.65 NE NE NE NE

TABLE IV Back Peripheral Optic Radii (Zonal Curvatures) for the following:
BCOR 7.0 to 8.8 in 0.1 steps
Zone Width 0.25 Zone Inner Diameters 6.0 to 11.5 in 0.5 steps
Axial Edge Lift Components 0.01 to 0.15 in 0.01 steps

```
FOR EDGE LIFT   0.01 ,   OPTIC DIAMETERS   6  -  6.5 ,   ZONAL CURVATURES ARE

 7.5  7.6  7.75  7.85  8  8.1  8.2  8.35  8.45  8.6  8.7  8.85  8.95  9.1  9.2  9.35  9.45  9.6  9.7

FOR EDGE LIFT   0.01 ,   OPTIC DIAMETERS   6.5  -  7 ,   ZONAL CURVATURES ARE

 7.4  7.55  7.65  7.8  7.9  8  8.15  8.25  8.4  8.5  8.6  8.75  8.85  9  9.1  9.25  9.35  9.5  9.6

FOR EDGE LIFT   0.01 ,   OPTIC DIAMETERS   7  -  7.5 ,   ZONAL CURVATURES ARE

 7.35  7.5  7.6  7.7  7.85  7.95  8.05  8.2  8.3  8.45  8.55  8.65  8.8  8.9  9.05  9.15  9.25  9.4  9.5

FOR EDGE LIFT   0.01 ,   OPTIC DIAMETERS   7.5  -  8 ,   ZONAL CURVATURES ARE

 7.3  7.45  7.55  7.65  7.8  7.9  8  8.15  8.25  8.35  8.5  8.6  8.7  8.85  8.95  9.05  9.2  9.3  9.45
```

```
FOR EDGE LIFT   0.01 ,   OPTIC DIAMETERS   8 - 8.5 ,   ZONAL CURVATURES ARE
 7.25  7.4  7.5  7.6  7.75  7.85  7.95  8.05  8.2  8.3  8.4  8.55  8.65  8.75  8.9  9  9.15  9.25  9.35

FOR EDGE LIFT   0.01 ,   OPTIC DIAMETERS   8.5 - 9 ,   ZONAL CURVATURES ARE
 7.25  7.35  7.45  7.55  7.7  7.8  7.9  8  8.15  8.25  8.35  8.5  8.6  8.7  8.85  8.95  9.05  9.2  9.3

FOR EDGE LIFT   0.01 ,   OPTIC DIAMETERS   9 - 9.5 ,   ZONAL CURVATURES ARE
 7.2  7.3  7.4  7.55  7.65  7.75  7.85  8  8.1  8.2  8.3  8.45  8.55  8.65  8.8  8.9  9  9.15  9.25

FOR EDGE LIFT   0.01 ,   OPTIC DIAMETERS   9.5 - 10 ,   ZONAL CURVATURES ARE
 7.15  7.25  7.4  7.5  7.6  7.7  7.85  7.95  8.05  8.15  8.3  8.4  8.5  8.6  8.75  8.85  8.95  9.1  9.2

FOR EDGE LIFT   0.01 ,   OPTIC DIAMETERS   10 - 10.5 ,   ZONAL CURVATURES ARE
 7.15  7.25  7.35  7.45  7.55  7.7  7.8  7.9  8  8.15  8.25  8.35  8.45  8.6  8.7  8.8  8.9  9.05  9.15

FOR EDGE LIFT   0.01 ,   OPTIC DIAMETERS   10.5 - 11 ,   ZONAL CURVATURES ARE
 7.1  7.2  7.3  7.45  7.55  7.65  7.75  7.85  8  8.1  8.2  8.3  8.45  8.55  8.65  8.75  8.9  9  9.1

FOR EDGE LIFT   0.01 ,   OPTIC DIAMETERS   11 - 11.5 ,   ZONAL CURVATURES ARE
 7.1  7.2  7.3  7.4  7.5  7.6  7.75  7.85  7.95  8.05  8.15  8.3  8.4  8.5  8.6  8.75  8.85  8.95  9.05

FOR EDGE LIFT   0.01 ,   OPTIC DIAMETERS   11.5 - 12 ,   ZONAL CURVATURES ARE
 7.05  7.15  7.25  7.4  7.5  7.6  7.7  7.8  7.9  8.05  8.15  8.25  8.35  8.45  8.6  8.7  8.8  8.9  9.05
```

```
FOR EDGE LIFT   0.02 ,   OPTIC DIAMETERS   6 - 6.5 ,    ZONAL CURVATURES ARE
 8.1  8.25  8.4  8.55  8.7  8.85  9  9.15  9.3  9.45  9.6  9.75  9.9  10.05  10.25  10.4  10.55  10.7  10.9

FOR EDGE LIFT   0.02 ,   OPTIC DIAMETERS   6.5 - 7 ,    ZONAL CURVATURES ARE
 7.95  8.05  8.2  8.35  8.5  8.65  8.8  8.95  9.1  9.25  9.4  9.55  9.7  9.85  10  10.15  10.3  10.45  10.6

FOR EDGE LIFT   0.02 ,   OPTIC DIAMETERS   7 - 7.5 ,    ZONAL CURVATURES ARE
 7.8  7.95  8.05  8.2  8.35  8.5  8.65  8.75  8.9  9.05  9.2  9.35  9.5  9.65  9.8  9.95  10.1  10.25  10.4

FOR EDGE LIFT   0.02 ,   OPTIC DIAMETERS   7.5 - 8 ,    ZONAL CURVATURES ARE
 7.7  7.8  7.95  8.1  8.2  8.35  8.5  8.65  8.75  8.9  9.05  9.2  9.35  9.5  9.6  9.75  9.9  10.05  10.2

FOR EDGE LIFT   0.02 ,   OPTIC DIAMETERS   8 - 8.5 ,    ZONAL CURVATURES ARE
 7.55  7.7  7.85  7.95  8.1  8.25  8.35  8.5  8.65  8.8  8.9  9.05  9.2  9.35  9.45  9.6  9.75  9.9  10.05

FOR EDGE LIFT   0.02 ,   OPTIC DIAMETERS   8.5 - 9 ,    ZONAL CURVATURES ARE
 7.5  7.6  7.75  7.85  8  8.15  8.25  8.4  8.55  8.65  8.8  8.95  9.05  9.2  9.35  9.5  9.6  9.75  9.9

FOR EDGE LIFT   0.02 ,   OPTIC DIAMETERS   9 - 9.5 ,    ZONAL CURVATURES ARE
 7.4  7.55  7.65  7.8  7.9  8.05  8.15  8.3  8.45  8.55  8.7  8.8  8.95  9.1  9.2  9.35  9.5  9.65  9.75

FOR EDGE LIFT   0.02 ,   OPTIC DIAMETERS   9.5 - 10 ,    ZONAL CURVATURES ARE
 7.35  7.45  7.6  7.7  7.85  7.95  8.1  8.2  8.35  8.45  8.6  8.75  8.85  9  9.1  9.25  9.4  9.5  9.65

FOR EDGE LIFT   0.02 ,   OPTIC DIAMETERS   10 - 10.5 ,    ZONAL CURVATURES ARE
 7.25  7.4  7.5  7.65  7.75  7.9  8  8.15  8.25  8.4  8.5  8.65  8.75  8.9  9  9.15  9.3  9.4  9.55

FOR EDGE LIFT   0.02 ,   OPTIC DIAMETERS   10.5 - 11 ,    ZONAL CURVATURES ARE
 7.2  7.35  7.45  7.55  7.7  7.8  7.95  8.05  8.2  8.3  8.45  8.55  8.7  8.8  8.95  9.05  9.2  9.3  9.45

FOR EDGE LIFT   0.02 ,   OPTIC DIAMETERS   11 - 11.5 ,    ZONAL CURVATURES ARE
 7.15  7.3  7.4  7.5  7.65  7.75  7.85  8  8.1  8.25  8.35  8.5  8.6  8.75  8.85  9  9.1  9.25  9.35

FOR EDGE LIFT   0.02 ,   OPTIC DIAMETERS   11.5 - 12 ,    ZONAL CURVATURES ARE
 7.1  7.25  7.35  7.45  7.6  7.7  7.8  7.95  8.05  8.2  8.3  8.4  8.55  8.65  8.8  8.9  9.05  9.15  9.3
```

FOR EDGE LIFT 0.03 , OPTIC DIAMETERS 6 - 6.5 , ZONAL CURVATURES ARE

8.8 9 9.2 9.35 9.55 9.75 9.95 10.15 10.35 10.55 10.75 10.95 11.15 11.35 11.55 11.75 12 12.2 12.4

FOR EDGE LIFT 0.03 , OPTIC DIAMETERS 6.5 - 7 , ZONAL CURVATURES ARE

8.55 8.7 8.9 9.05 9.25 9.4 9.6 9.8 9.95 10.15 10.35 10.55 10.7 10.9 11.1 11.3 11.5 11.7 11.9

FOR EDGE LIFT 0.03 , OPTIC DIAMETERS 7 - 7.5 , ZONAL CURVATURES ARE

8.3 8.45 8.65 8.8 8.95 9.15 9.3 9.5 9.65 9.85 10 10.2 10.35 10.55 10.75 10.95 11.1 11.3 11.5

FOR EDGE LIFT 0.03 , OPTIC DIAMETERS 7.5 - 8 , ZONAL CURVATURES ARE

8.1 8.25 8.4 8.6 8.75 8.9 9.05 9.25 9.4 9.55 9.75 9.9 10.1 10.25 10.45 10.6 10.8 10.95 11.15

FOR EDGE LIFT 0.03 , OPTIC DIAMETERS 8 - 8.5 , ZONAL CURVATURES ARE

7.95 8.1 8.25 8.4 8.55 8.7 8.85 9 9.2 9.35 9.5 9.65 9.85 10 10.15 10.35 10.5 10.7 10.85

FOR EDGE LIFT 0.03 , OPTIC DIAMETERS 8.5 - 9 , ZONAL CURVATURES ARE

7.75 7.9 8.05 8.2 8.35 8.5 8.65 8.85 9 9.15 9.3 9.45 9.6 9.8 9.95 10.1 10.25 10.45 10.6

FOR EDGE LIFT 0.03 , OPTIC DIAMETERS 9 - 9.5 , ZONAL CURVATURES ARE

7.65 7.8 7.95 8.05 8.2 8.35 8.5 8.65 8.8 8.95 9.1 9.25 9.45 9.6 9.75 9.9 10.05 10.2 10.4

FOR EDGE LIFT 0.03 , OPTIC DIAMETERS 9.5 - 10 , ZONAL CURVATURES ARE

7.5 7.65 7.8 7.95 8.1 8.25 8.35 8.5 8.65 8.8 8.95 9.1 9.25 9.4 9.55 9.7 9.85 10 10.2

FOR EDGE LIFT 0.03 , OPTIC DIAMETERS 10 - 10.5 , ZONAL CURVATURES ARE

7.4 7.55 7.7 7.85 7.95 8.1 8.25 8.4 8.55 8.65 8.8 8.95 9.1 9.25 9.4 9.55 9.7 9.85 10

FOR EDGE LIFT 0.03 , OPTIC DIAMETERS 10.5 - 11 , ZONAL CURVATURES ARE

7.35 7.45 7.6 7.75 7.85 8 8.15 8.25 8.4 8.55 8.7 8.85 8.95 9.1 9.25 9.4 9.55 9.7 9.85

FOR EDGE LIFT 0.03 , OPTIC DIAMETERS 11 - 11.5 , ZONAL CURVATURES ARE

7.25 7.4 7.5 7.65 7.75 7.9 8.05 8.15 8.3 8.45 8.6 8.7 8.85 9 9.15 9.25 9.4 9.55 9.7

FOR EDGE LIFT 0.03 , OPTIC DIAMETERS 11.5 - 12 , ZONAL CURVATURES ARE

7.2 7.3 7.45 7.55 7.7 7.8 7.95 8.05 8.2 8.35 8.45 8.6 8.75 8.9 9 9.15 9.3 9.45 9.6

```
FOR EDGE LIFT    0.04 ,    OPTIC DIAMETERS    6  -  6.5 ,     ZONAL CURVATURES ARE
 9.75  9.95  10.2  10.45  10.7  10.95  11.2  11.45  11.7  11.95  12.25  12.5  12.8  13.05  13.35  13.65  13.95  14.25  14.55

FOR EDGE LIFT    0.04 ,    OPTIC DIAMETERS    6.5  -  7 ,     ZONAL CURVATURES ARE
 9.3  9.5  9.7  9.95  10.15  10.4  10.6  10.85  11.05  11.3  11.55  11.8  12.05  12.3  12.55  12.85  13.1  13.35  13.65

FOR EDGE LIFT    0.04 ,    OPTIC DIAMETERS    7  -  7.5 ,     ZONAL CURVATURES ARE
 8.9  9.1  9.3  9.5  9.7  9.95  10.15  10.35  10.55  10.8  11  11.25  11.5  11.7  11.95  12.2  12.45  12.7  12.95

FOR EDGE LIFT    0.04 ,    OPTIC DIAMETERS    7.5  -  8 ,     ZONAL CURVATURES ARE
 8.6  8.8  8.95  9.15  9.35  9.55  9.75  9.95  10.15  10.35  10.6  10.8  11  11.2  11.45  11.65  11.9  12.1  12.35

FOR EDGE LIFT    0.04 ,    OPTIC DIAMETERS    8  -  8.5 ,     ZONAL CURVATURES ARE
 8.35  8.5  8.7  8.85  9.05  9.25  9.45  9.6  9.8  10  10.2  10.4  10.6  10.8  11  11.25  11.45  11.65  11.85

FOR EDGE LIFT    0.04 ,    OPTIC DIAMETERS    8.5  -  9 ,     ZONAL CURVATURES ARE
 8.1  8.3  8.45  8.6  8.8  8.95  9.15  9.35  9.5  9.7  9.9  10.1  10.25  10.45  10.65  10.85  11.05  11.25  11.45

FOR EDGE LIFT    0.04 ,    OPTIC DIAMETERS    9  -  9.5 ,     ZONAL CURVATURES ARE
 7.9  8.05  8.25  8.4  8.55  8.75  8.9  9.1  9.25  9.45  9.6  9.8  10  10.15  10.35  10.55  10.7  10.9  11.1

FOR EDGE LIFT    0.04 ,    OPTIC DIAMETERS    9.5  -  10 ,     ZONAL CURVATURES ARE
 7.75  7.9  8.05  8.2  8.4  8.55  8.7  8.85  9.05  9.2  9.4  9.55  9.7  9.9  10.1  10.25  10.45  10.6  10.8

FOR EDGE LIFT    0.04 ,    OPTIC DIAMETERS    10  -  10.5 ,     ZONAL CURVATURES ARE
 7.6  7.75  7.9  8.05  8.2  8.35  8.5  8.7  8.85  9  9.15  9.35  9.5  9.65  9.85  10  10.2  10.35  10.55

FOR EDGE LIFT    0.04 ,    OPTIC DIAMETERS    10.5  -  11 ,     ZONAL CURVATURES ARE
 7.45  7.6  7.75  7.9  8.05  8.2  8.35  8.5  8.65  8.8  9  9.15  9.3  9.45  9.65  9.8  9.95  10.15  10.3

FOR EDGE LIFT    0.04 ,    OPTIC DIAMETERS    11  -  11.5 ,     ZONAL CURVATURES ARE
 7.35  7.5  7.65  7.75  7.9  8.05  8.2  8.35  8.5  8.65  8.8  8.95  9.1  9.3  9.45  9.6  9.75  9.95  10.1

FOR EDGE LIFT    0.04 ,    OPTIC DIAMETERS    11.5  -  12 ,     ZONAL CURVATURES ARE
 7.25  7.4  7.5  7.65  7.8  7.95  8.1  8.2  8.35  8.5  8.65  8.8  8.95  9.1  9.25  9.45  9.6  9.75  9.9
```

FOR EDGE LIFT 0.05 , OPTIC DIAMETERS 6 - 6.5 , ZONAL CURVATURES ARE

10.9 11.2 11.5 11.85 12.15 12.5 12.85 13.2 13.55 13.9 14.25 14.65 15.05 15.45 15.85 16.3 16.75 17.2 17.65

FOR EDGE LIFT 0.05 , OPTIC DIAMETERS 6.5 - 7 , ZONAL CURVATURES ARE

10.2 10.45 10.75 11.05 11.3 11.6 11.9 12.2 12.5 12.85 13.15 13.5 13.85 14.15 14.55 14.9 15.25 15.65 16.05

FOR EDGE LIFT 0.05 , OPTIC DIAMETERS 7 - 7.5 , ZONAL CURVATURES ARE

9.65 9.9 10.15 10.4 10.65 10.9 11.2 11.45 11.75 12 12.3 12.6 12.9 13.2 13.5 13.85 14.15 14.5 14.85

FOR EDGE LIFT 0.05 , OPTIC DIAMETERS 7.5 - 8 , ZONAL CURVATURES ARE

9.2 9.4 9.65 9.9 10.1 10.35 10.6 10.85 11.1 11.35 11.6 11.9 12.15 12.45 12.7 13 13.3 13.6 13.9

FOR EDGE LIFT 0.05 , OPTIC DIAMETERS 8 - 8.5 , ZONAL CURVATURES ARE

8.8 9 9.25 9.45 9.65 9.9 10.1 10.35 10.6 10.8 11.05 11.3 11.55 11.8 12.05 12.35 12.6 12.85 13.15

FOR EDGE LIFT 0.05 , OPTIC DIAMETERS 8.5 - 9 , ZONAL CURVATURES ARE

8.5 8.7 8.9 9.1 9.3 9.5 9.7 9.95 10.15 10.35 10.6 10.8 11.05 11.3 11.55 11.75 12 12.25 12.5

FOR EDGE LIFT 0.05 , OPTIC DIAMETERS 9 - 9.5 , ZONAL CURVATURES ARE

8.2 8.4 8.6 8.8 9 9.2 9.4 9.6 9.8 10 10.2 10.4 10.65 10.85 11.05 11.3 11.55 11.75 12

FOR EDGE LIFT 0.05 , OPTIC DIAMETERS 9.5 - 10 , ZONAL CURVATURES ARE

8 8.15 8.35 8.5 8.7 8.9 9.1 9.25 9.45 9.65 9.85 10.05 10.25 10.45 10.7 10.9 11.1 11.35 11.55

FOR EDGE LIFT 0.05 , OPTIC DIAMETERS 10 - 10.5 , ZONAL CURVATURES ARE

7.8 7.95 8.1 8.3 8.45 8.65 8.8 9 9.2 9.4 9.55 9.75 9.95 10.15 10.35 10.55 10.75 10.95 11.15

FOR EDGE LIFT 0.05 , OPTIC DIAMETERS 10.5 - 11 , ZONAL CURVATURES ARE

7.6 7.75 7.95 8.1 8.25 8.45 8.6 8.75 8.95 9.15 9.3 9.5 9.7 9.85 10.05 10.25 10.45 10.65 10.85

FOR EDGE LIFT 0.05 , OPTIC DIAMETERS 11 - 11.5 , ZONAL CURVATURES ARE

7.45 7.6 7.75 7.9 8.1 8.25 8.4 8.55 8.75 8.9 9.1 9.25 9.45 9.6 9.8 9.95 10.15 10.35 10.55

FOR EDGE LIFT 0.05 , OPTIC DIAMETERS 11.5 - 12 , ZONAL CURVATURES ARE

7.3 7.45 7.6 7.75 7.9 8.05 8.25 8.4 8.55 8.7 8.9 9.05 9.2 9.4 9.55 9.75 9.9 10.1 10.3

```
FOR EDGE LIFT   6.00000E-2 ,   OPTIC DIAMETERS   6 - 6.5 ,   ZONAL CURVATURES ARE
 12.45  12.85  13.3  13.75  14.2  14.65  15.15  15.6  16.15  16.7  17.25  17.8  18.4  19.05  19.7  20.35  21.05  21.8  22.55

FOR EDGE LIFT   6.00000E-2 ,   OPTIC DIAMETERS   6.5 - 7 ,   ZONAL CURVATURES ARE
 11.4  11.75  12.1  12.45  12.85  13.2  13.6  14.05  14.45  14.9  15.35  15.8  16.3  16.8  17.3  17.85  18.4  18.95  19.55

FOR EDGE LIFT   6.00000E-2 ,   OPTIC DIAMETERS   7 - 7.5 ,   ZONAL CURVATURES ARE
 10.55  10.85  11.2  11.5  11.85  12.15  12.5  12.85  13.25  13.6  14  14.4  14.8  15.2  15.65  16.05  16.5  17  17.45

FOR EDGE LIFT   6.00000E-2 ,   OPTIC DIAMETERS   7.5 - 8 ,   ZONAL CURVATURES ARE
 9.9  10.2  10.45  10.75  11.05  11.35  11.65  11.95  12.3  12.6  12.95  13.3  13.65  14  14.35  14.75  15.15  15.55  15.95

FOR EDGE LIFT   6.00000E-2 ,   OPTIC DIAMETERS   8 - 8.5 ,   ZONAL CURVATURES ARE
 9.4  9.65  9.9  10.15  10.4  10.7  10.95  11.25  11.55  11.8  12.1  12.45  12.75  13.05  13.4  13.7  14.05  14.4  14.8

FOR EDGE LIFT   6.00000E-2 ,   OPTIC DIAMETERS   8.5 - 9 ,   ZONAL CURVATURES ARE
 8.95  9.15  9.4  9.65  9.9  10.15  10.4  10.65  10.9  11.2  11.45  11.75  12  12.3  12.6  12.9  13.2  13.5  13.85

FOR EDGE LIFT   6.00000E-2 ,   OPTIC DIAMETERS   9 - 9.5 ,   ZONAL CURVATURES ARE
 8.55  8.8  9  9.25  9.45  9.7  9.9  10.15  10.4  10.65  10.9  11.15  11.4  11.7  11.95  12.25  12.5  12.8  13.1

FOR EDGE LIFT   6.00000E-2 ,   OPTIC DIAMETERS   9.5 - 10 ,   ZONAL CURVATURES ARE
 8.25  8.45  8.65  8.85  9.1  9.3  9.5  9.75  9.95  10.2  10.45  10.65  10.9  11.15  11.4  11.65  11.9  12.2  12.45

FOR EDGE LIFT   6.00000E-2 ,   OPTIC DIAMETERS   10 - 10.5 ,   ZONAL CURVATURES ARE
 8  8.2  8.35  8.55  8.75  8.95  9.15  9.4  9.6  9.8  10.05  10.25  10.5  10.7  10.95  11.2  11.4  11.65  11.9

FOR EDGE LIFT   6.00000E-2 ,   OPTIC DIAMETERS   10.5 - 11 ,   ZONAL CURVATURES ARE
 7.75  7.95  8.1  8.3  8.5  8.7  8.9  9.05  9.25  9.5  9.7  9.9  10.1  10.3  10.55  10.75  11  11.2  11.45

FOR EDGE LIFT   6.00000E-2 ,   OPTIC DIAMETERS   11 - 11.5 ,   ZONAL CURVATURES ARE
 7.55  7.75  7.9  8.1  8.25  8.45  8.6  8.8  9  9.2  9.4  9.6  9.8  10  10.2  10.4  10.6  10.85  11.05

FOR EDGE LIFT   6.00000E-2 ,   OPTIC DIAMETERS   11.5 - 12 ,   ZONAL CURVATURES ARE
 7.4  7.55  7.7  7.9  8.05  8.2  8.4  8.55  8.75  8.95  9.1  9.3  9.5  9.7  9.9  10.1  10.3  10.5  10.7
```

```
FOR EDGE LIFT   0.07 ,   OPTIC DIAMETERS   6 - 6.5 ,   ZONAL CURVATURES ARE
14.6  15.2  15.8  16.45  17.1  17.8  18.5  19.3  20.1  20.95  21.85  22.8  23.85  24.9  26.05  27.25  28.55  29.95  31.45

FOR EDGE LIFT   0.07 ,   OPTIC DIAMETERS   6.5 - 7 ,   ZONAL CURVATURES ARE
12.95  13.4  13.85  14.4  14.9  15.45  16  16.6  17.2  17.85  18.5  19.2  19.95  20.7  21.5  22.35  23.25  24.2  25.15

FOR EDGE LIFT   0.07 ,   OPTIC DIAMETERS   7 - 7.5 ,   ZONAL CURVATURES ARE
11.7  12.1  12.5  12.9  13.35  13.8  14.25  14.75  15.25  15.75  16.3  16.85  17.4  18  18.6  19.25  19.95  20.65  21.35

FOR EDGE LIFT   0.07 ,   OPTIC DIAMETERS   7.5 - 8 ,   ZONAL CURVATURES ARE
10.8  11.15  11.5  11.85  12.2  12.6  13  13.4  13.8  14.25  14.7  15.15  15.6  16.1  16.6  17.15  17.65  18.25  18.8

FOR EDGE LIFT   0.07 ,   OPTIC DIAMETERS   8 - 8.5 ,   ZONAL CURVATURES ARE
10.05  10.35  10.65  11  11.3  11.65  12  12.35  12.7  13.1  13.45  13.85  14.25  14.7  15.1  15.55  16  16.5  16.95

FOR EDGE LIFT   0.07 ,   OPTIC DIAMETERS   8.5 - 9 ,   ZONAL CURVATURES ARE
9.45  9.75  10  10.3  10.6  10.9  11.2  11.5  11.85  12.15  12.5  12.85  13.2  13.6  13.95  14.35  14.75  15.15  15.55

FOR EDGE LIFT   0.07 ,   OPTIC DIAMETERS   9 - 9.5 ,   ZONAL CURVATURES ARE
9  9.25  9.5  9.75  10  10.3  10.55  10.85  11.15  11.45  11.75  12.05  12.35  12.7  13.05  13.35  13.7  14.1  14.45

FOR EDGE LIFT   0.07 ,   OPTIC DIAMETERS   9.5 - 10 ,   ZONAL CURVATURES ARE
8.6  8.8  9.05  9.3  9.5  9.75  10.05  10.3  10.55  10.8  11.1  11.4  11.7  11.95  12.25  12.6  12.9  13.2  13.55

FOR EDGE LIFT   0.07 ,   OPTIC DIAMETERS   10 - 10.5 ,   ZONAL CURVATURES ARE
8.25  8.45  8.65  8.9  9.1  9.35  9.6  9.8  10.05  10.3  10.55  10.85  11.1  11.35  11.65  11.95  12.2  12.5  12.8

FOR EDGE LIFT   0.07 ,   OPTIC DIAMETERS   10.5 - 11 ,   ZONAL CURVATURES ARE
7.95  8.15  8.35  8.55  8.75  8.95  9.2  9.4  9.65  9.9  10.1  10.35  10.6  10.85  11.1  11.35  11.65  11.9  12.2

FOR EDGE LIFT   0.07 ,   OPTIC DIAMETERS   11 - 11.5 ,   ZONAL CURVATURES ARE
7.7  7.9  8.05  8.25  8.45  8.65  8.85  9.05  9.3  9.5  9.7  9.95  10.2  10.4  10.65  10.9  11.15  11.4  11.65

FOR EDGE LIFT   0.07 ,   OPTIC DIAMETERS   11.5 - 12 ,   ZONAL CURVATURES ARE
7.5  7.65  7.85  8  8.2  8.4  8.6  8.8  9  9.2  9.4  9.6  9.8  10.05  10.25  10.5  10.7  10.95  11.2
```

FOR EDGE LIFT 0.08 , OPTIC DIAMETERS 6 - 6.5 , ZONAL CURVATURES ARE

17.75 18.6 19.55 20.55 21.65 22.8 24.05 25.35 26.8 28.4 30.1 31.95 34 36.25 38.8 41.55 44.7 48.25 52.25

FOR EDGE LIFT 0.08 , OPTIC DIAMETERS 6.5 - 7 , ZONAL CURVATURES ARE

15.05 15.7 16.35 17.1 17.85 18.65 19.5 20.4 21.35 22.35 23.45 24.6 25.85 27.2 28.6 30.15 31.8 33.6 35.55

FOR EDGE LIFT 0.08 , OPTIC DIAMETERS 7 - 7.5 , ZONAL CURVATURES ARE

13.2 13.7 14.25 14.8 15.4 16.05 16.65 17.35 18.05 18.8 19.6 20.4 21.25 22.2 23.15 24.2 25.3 26.45 27.65

FOR EDGE LIFT 0.08 , OPTIC DIAMETERS 7.5 - 8 , ZONAL CURVATURES ARE

11.9 12.3 12.75 13.2 13.7 14.2 14.7 15.25 15.85 16.4 17 17.65 18.35 19.05 19.75 20.5 21.3 22.15 23.05

FOR EDGE LIFT 0.08 , OPTIC DIAMETERS 8 - 8.5 , ZONAL CURVATURES ARE

10.9 11.25 11.65 12.05 12.45 12.85 13.3 13.75 14.2 14.7 15.2 15.7 16.25 16.85 17.4 18 18.65 19.3 20

FOR EDGE LIFT 0.08 , OPTIC DIAMETERS 8.5 - 9 , ZONAL CURVATURES ARE

10.1 10.4 10.75 11.1 11.45 11.8 12.2 12.6 13 13.4 13.85 14.3 14.75 15.2 15.7 16.2 16.75 17.25 17.85

FOR EDGE LIFT 0.08 , OPTIC DIAMETERS 9 - 9.5 , ZONAL CURVATURES ARE

9.45 9.75 10.05 10.35 10.65 11 11.35 11.65 12.05 12.4 12.75 13.15 13.55 13.95 14.4 14.8 15.25 15.7 16.2

FOR EDGE LIFT 0.08 , OPTIC DIAMETERS 9.5 - 10 , ZONAL CURVATURES ARE

8.95 9.2 9.45 9.75 10.05 10.3 10.6 10.95 11.25 11.55 11.9 12.25 12.6 12.95 13.35 13.7 14.1 14.5 14.95

FOR EDGE LIFT 0.08 , OPTIC DIAMETERS 10 - 10.5 , ZONAL CURVATURES ARE

8.5 8.75 9 9.25 9.5 9.75 10.05 10.3 10.6 10.9 11.2 11.5 11.85 12.15 12.5 12.8 13.15 13.55 13.9

FOR EDGE LIFT 0.08 , OPTIC DIAMETERS 10.5 - 11 , ZONAL CURVATURES ARE

8.15 8.35 8.6 8.8 9.05 9.3 9.55 9.8 10.05 10.35 10.6 10.9 11.2 11.5 11.8 12.1 12.4 12.75 13.05

FOR EDGE LIFT 0.08 , OPTIC DIAMETERS 11 - 11.5 , ZONAL CURVATURES ARE

7.85 8.05 8.25 8.45 8.7 8.9 9.15 9.35 9.6 9.85 10.1 10.35 10.65 10.9 11.2 11.45 11.75 12.05 12.35

FOR EDGE LIFT 0.08 , OPTIC DIAMETERS 11.5 - 12 , ZONAL CURVATURES ARE

7.6 7.75 7.95 8.15 8.35 8.55 8.8 9 9.25 9.45 9.7 9.95 10.15 10.4 10.7 10.95 11.2 11.5 11.75

```
FOR EDGE LIFT    0.09 ,    OPTIC DIAMETERS    6  -  6.5 ,     ZONAL CURVATURES ARE
 22.7  24.2  25.85  27.65  29.65  31.9  34.4  37.25  40.5  44.25  48.6  53.75  59.85  67.3 NE  NE  NE  NE  NE

FOR EDGE LIFT    0.09 ,    OPTIC DIAMETERS    6.5  -  7 ,     ZONAL CURVATURES ARE
 18.05  19  20.05  21.15  22.35  23.7  25.1  26.65  28.3  30.15  32.2  34.45  36.95  39.8  42.95  46.55  50.7  55.45  61.1

FOR EDGE LIFT    0.09 ,    OPTIC DIAMETERS    7  -  7.5 ,     ZONAL CURVATURES ARE
 15.2  15.9  16.65  17.45  18.3  19.2  20.15  21.2  22.25  23.45  24.7  26.05  27.5  29.1  30.8  32.7  34.75  37  39.5

FOR EDGE LIFT    0.09 ,    OPTIC DIAMETERS    7.5  -  8 ,     ZONAL CURVATURES ARE
 13.3  13.85  14.45  15.05  15.7  16.35  17.1  17.85  18.65  19.5  20.35  21.3  22.3  23.4  24.5  25.75  27.05  28.45  29.95

FOR EDGE LIFT    0.09 ,    OPTIC DIAMETERS    8  -  8.5 ,     ZONAL CURVATURES ARE
 11.9  12.35  12.85  13.35  13.85  14.4  15  15.6  16.2  16.85  17.55  18.25  19  19.8  20.65  21.55  22.45  23.45  24.5

FOR EDGE LIFT    0.09 ,    OPTIC DIAMETERS    8.5  -  9 ,     ZONAL CURVATURES ARE
 10.85  11.25  11.65  12.05  12.5  12.95  13.45  13.95  14.45  15  15.55  16.1  16.75  17.35  18  18.7  19.45  20.2  21

FOR EDGE LIFT    0.09 ,    OPTIC DIAMETERS    9  -  9.5 ,     ZONAL CURVATURES ARE
 10  10.35  10.7  11.1  11.45  11.85  12.25  12.7  13.1  13.6  14.05  14.55  15.05  15.55  16.1  16.7  17.25  17.9  18.5

FOR EDGE LIFT    0.09 ,    OPTIC DIAMETERS    9.5  -  10 ,     ZONAL CURVATURES ARE
 9.35  9.65  9.95  10.3  10.65  11  11.35  11.7  12.1  12.5  12.9  13.3  13.75  14.2  14.65  15.15  15.65  16.15  16.7

FOR EDGE LIFT    0.09 ,    OPTIC DIAMETERS    10  -  10.5 ,     ZONAL CURVATURES ARE
 8.8  9.1  9.35  9.65  9.95  10.25  10.6  10.9  11.25  11.6  11.95  12.3  12.7  13.1  13.5  13.9  14.35  14.8  15.25

FOR EDGE LIFT    0.09 ,    OPTIC DIAMETERS    10.5  -  11 ,     ZONAL CURVATURES ARE
 8.35  8.6  8.85  9.15  9.4  9.7  9.95  10.25  10.55  10.85  11.2  11.5  11.85  12.2  12.55  12.95  13.3  13.7  14.1

FOR EDGE LIFT    0.09 ,    OPTIC DIAMETERS    11  -  11.5 ,     ZONAL CURVATURES ARE
 8  8.2  8.45  8.7  8.95  9.2  9.45  9.7  10  10.25  10.55  10.85  11.15  11.5  11.8  12.15  12.5  12.85  13.2

FOR EDGE LIFT    0.09 ,    OPTIC DIAMETERS    11.5  -  12 ,     ZONAL CURVATURES ARE
 7.7  7.9  8.1  8.3  8.55  8.8  9  9.25  9.5  9.75  10.05  10.3  10.6  10.85  11.15  11.45  11.75  12.1  12.4
```

FOR EDGE LIFT 0.1 , OPTIC DIAMETERS 6 - 6.5 , ZONAL CURVATURES ARE

31.7 34.75 38.3 42.45 47.45 53.55 61.15 NE NE NE NE NE NE NE NE NE NE NE NE

FOR EDGE LIFT 0.1 , OPTIC DIAMETERS 6.5 - 7 , ZONAL CURVATURES ARE

22.7 24.25 26 28 30.15 32.6 35.4 38.6 42.3 46.6 51.7 57.85 NE NE NE NE NE NE NE

FOR EDGE LIFT 0.1 , OPTIC DIAMETERS 7 - 7.5 , ZONAL CURVATURES ARE

18 19.05 20.15 21.35 22.65 24.1 25.65 27.35 29.25 31.3 33.65 36.25 39.15 42.5 46.35 50.8 56 62.15 NE

FOR EDGE LIFT 0.1 , OPTIC DIAMETERS 7.5 - 8 , ZONAL CURVATURES ARE

15.15 15.9 16.7 17.55 18.45 19.4 20.45 21.6 22.8 24.1 25.5 27 28.7 30.5 32.5 34.7 37.2 39.9 43

FOR EDGE LIFT 0.1 , OPTIC DIAMETERS 8 - 8.5 , ZONAL CURVATURES ARE

13.2 13.75 14.4 15.05 15.75 16.45 17.25 18.05 18.95 19.85 20.85 21.9 23 24.2 25.5 26.9 28.4 30.05 31.8

FOR EDGE LIFT 0.1 , OPTIC DIAMETERS 8.5 - 9 , ZONAL CURVATURES ARE

11.75 12.25 12.75 13.3 13.85 14.4 15.05 15.7 16.35 17.05 17.8 18.6 19.45 20.35 21.25 22.25 23.3 24.45 25.65

FOR EDGE LIFT 0.1 , OPTIC DIAMETERS 9 - 9.5 , ZONAL CURVATURES ARE

10.7 11.1 11.5 11.95 12.45 12.9 13.4 13.95 14.5 15.1 15.7 16.3 16.95 17.65 18.4 19.15 19.95 20.85 21.7

FOR EDGE LIFT 0.1 , OPTIC DIAMETERS 9.5 - 10 , ZONAL CURVATURES ARE

9.85 10.2 10.55 10.95 11.35 11.75 12.2 12.65 13.1 13.6 14.1 14.6 15.15 15.75 16.35 16.95 17.6 18.3 19

FOR EDGE LIFT 0.1 , OPTIC DIAMETERS 10 - 10.5 , ZONAL CURVATURES ARE

9.15 9.45 9.8 10.15 10.5 10.85 11.2 11.6 12 12.45 12.85 13.3 13.75 14.25 14.75 15.3 15.85 16.4 17

FOR EDGE LIFT 0.1 , OPTIC DIAMETERS 10.5 - 11 , ZONAL CURVATURES ARE

8.6 8.9 9.2 9.5 9.8 10.1 10.45 10.8 11.15 11.5 11.9 12.25 12.7 13.1 13.55 14 14.45 14.95 15.45

FOR EDGE LIFT 0.1 , OPTIC DIAMETERS 11 - 11.5 , ZONAL CURVATURES ARE

8.15 8.4 8.65 8.95 9.2 9.5 9.8 10.1 10.4 10.75 11.1 11.45 11.8 12.15 12.55 12.95 13.35 13.75 14.2

FOR EDGE LIFT 0.1 , OPTIC DIAMETERS 11.5 - 12 , ZONAL CURVATURES ARE

7.8 8 8.25 8.5 8.75 9 9.25 9.55 9.85 10.1 10.4 10.75 11.05 11.4 11.75 12.1 12.45 12.8 13.2

```
FOR EDGE LIFT   0.11 ,   OPTIC DIAMETERS   6 - 6.5 ,   ZONAL CURVATURES ARE
 53.05  62.2 NE  NE  NE  NE  NE  NE  NE  NE  NE  NE  NE  NE  NE  NE  NE  NE  NE

FOR EDGE LIFT   0.11 ,   OPTIC DIAMETERS   6.5 - 7 ,   ZONAL CURVATURES ARE
 30.75  33.75  37.35  41.55  46.6  52.85  60.65 NE  NE  NE  NE  NE  NE  NE  NE  NE  NE  NE  NE

FOR EDGE LIFT   0.11 ,   OPTIC DIAMETERS   7 - 7.5 ,   ZONAL CURVATURES ARE
 22.2  23.8  25.65  27.65  29.9  32.5  35.45  38.85  42.8  47.5  53.1  60 NE  NE  NE  NE  NE  NE  NE

FOR EDGE LIFT   0.11 ,   OPTIC DIAMETERS   7.5 - 8 ,   ZONAL CURVATURES ARE
 17.65  18.7  19.9  21.15  22.5  24  25.65  27.45  29.5  31.75  34.3  37.15  40.4  44.2  48.55  53.75  59.9 NE  NE

FOR EDGE LIFT   0.11 ,   OPTIC DIAMETERS   8 - 8.5 ,   ZONAL CURVATURES ARE
 14.85  15.6  16.45  17.35  18.3  19.3  20.4  21.6  22.9  24.3  25.8  27.45  29.3  31.3  33.55  36.05  38.85  42.05  45.65

FOR EDGE LIFT   0.11 ,   OPTIC DIAMETERS   8.5 - 9 ,   ZONAL CURVATURES ARE
 12.9  13.5  14.15  14.8  15.55  16.3  17.15  18  18.9  19.9  20.95  22.1  23.3  24.65  26.05  27.6  29.3  31.15  33.15

FOR EDGE LIFT   0.11 ,   OPTIC DIAMETERS   9 - 9.5 ,   ZONAL CURVATURES ARE
 11.45  11.95  12.5  13.05  13.6  14.25  14.85  15.55  16.25  17  17.8  18.65  19.55  20.55  21.55  22.65  23.8  25.05  26.4

FOR EDGE LIFT   0.11 ,   OPTIC DIAMETERS   9.5 - 10 ,   ZONAL CURVATURES ARE
 10.4  10.8  11.25  11.7  12.2  12.7  13.25  13.8  14.35  14.95  15.6  16.3  17  17.75  18.5  19.35  20.25  21.15  22.15

FOR EDGE LIFT   0.11 ,   OPTIC DIAMETERS   10 - 10.5 ,   ZONAL CURVATURES ARE
 9.55  9.9  10.3  10.7  11.1  11.55  11.95  12.45  12.95  13.45  13.95  14.5  15.1  15.7  16.35  17  17.7  18.45  19.25

FOR EDGE LIFT   0.11 ,   OPTIC DIAMETERS   10.5 - 11 ,   ZONAL CURVATURES ARE
 8.9  9.2  9.55  9.9  10.25  10.6  11  11.4  11.8  12.25  12.7  13.15  13.65  14.15  14.7  15.25  15.85  16.45  17.1

FOR EDGE LIFT   0.11 ,   OPTIC DIAMETERS   11 - 11.5 ,   ZONAL CURVATURES ARE
 8.35  8.65  8.9  9.2  9.55  9.85  10.2  10.55  10.9  11.3  11.7  12.1  12.5  12.95  13.4  13.9  14.4  14.9  15.45

FOR EDGE LIFT   0.11 ,   OPTIC DIAMETERS   11.5 - 12 ,   ZONAL CURVATURES ARE
 7.9  8.15  8.4  8.7  8.95  9.25  9.55  9.85  10.2  10.5  10.85  11.25  11.6  12  12.4  12.8  13.25  13.65  14.15
```

FOR EDGE LIFT 0.12 , OPTIC DIAMETERS 6 - 6.5 , ZONAL CURVATURES ARE

NE NE NE NE NE NE NE NE NE NE NE NE NE NE NE NE NE NE NE

FOR EDGE LIFT 0.12 , OPTIC DIAMETERS 6.5 - 7 , ZONAL CURVATURES ARE

48 55.95 66.55 81.35 NE NE NE NE NE NE NE NE NE NE NE NE NE NE NE

FOR EDGE LIFT 0.12 , OPTIC DIAMETERS 7 - 7.5 , ZONAL CURVATURES ARE

29.1 32 35.4 39.45 44.35 50.3 57.85 67.55 80.65 NE NE NE NE NE NE NE NE NE NE

FOR EDGE LIFT 0.12 , OPTIC DIAMETERS 7.5 - 8 , ZONAL CURVATURES ARE

21.3 22.9 24.7 26.75 29 31.6 34.55 38 42.05 46.85 52.65 59.85 68.95 80.75 NE NE NE NE NE

FOR EDGE LIFT 0.12 , OPTIC DIAMETERS 8 - 8.5 , ZONAL CURVATURES ARE

17.05 18.1 19.25 20.55 21.9 23.45 25.15 27 29.1 31.45 34.1 37.1 40.6 44.6 49.4 55.05 61.95 70.5 81.4

FOR EDGE LIFT 0.12 , OPTIC DIAMETERS 8.5 - 9 , ZONAL CURVATURES ARE

14.3 15.1 15.95 16.85 17.8 18.85 20 21.2 22.55 24 25.6 27.35 29.3 31.45 33.85 36.6 39.65 43.15 47.2

FOR EDGE LIFT 0.12 , OPTIC DIAMETERS 9 - 9.5 , ZONAL CURVATURES ARE

12.45 13.05 13.7 14.4 15.15 15.9 16.75 17.65 18.6 19.65 20.75 21.95 23.25 24.6 26.15 27.8 29.65 31.65 33.85

FOR EDGE LIFT 0.12 , OPTIC DIAMETERS 9.5 - 10 , ZONAL CURVATURES ARE

11.05 11.55 12.1 12.65 13.25 13.85 14.5 15.2 15.95 16.75 17.55 18.45 19.4 20.4 21.5 22.65 23.9 25.25 26.7

FOR EDGE LIFT 0.12 , OPTIC DIAMETERS 10 - 10.5 , ZONAL CURVATURES ARE

10 10.45 10.9 11.35 11.85 12.35 12.9 13.45 14.05 14.65 15.35 16.05 16.75 17.55 18.4 19.25 20.2 21.2 22.25

FOR EDGE LIFT 0.12 , OPTIC DIAMETERS 10.5 - 11 , ZONAL CURVATURES ARE

9.2 9.55 9.95 10.35 10.75 11.2 11.65 12.1 12.6 13.15 13.65 14.25 14.85 15.5 16.15 16.85 17.6 18.35 19.2

FOR EDGE LIFT 0.12 , OPTIC DIAMETERS 11 - 11.5 , ZONAL CURVATURES ARE

8.55 8.85 9.2 9.55 9.9 10.25 10.65 11.05 11.5 11.95 12.4 12.9 13.4 13.9 14.45 15.05 15.65 16.3 16.95

FOR EDGE LIFT 0.12 , OPTIC DIAMETERS 11.5 - 12 , ZONAL CURVATURES ARE

8.05 8.35 8.6 8.9 9.2 9.55 9.9 10.25 10.6 11 11.4 11.8 12.25 12.7 13.15 13.65 14.15 14.7 15.25

FOR EDGE LIFT 0.13 , OPTIC DIAMETERS 6 - 6.5 , ZONAL CURVATURES ARE

NE NE NE NE NE NE NE NE NE NE NE NE NE NE NE NE NE NE NE

FOR EDGE LIFT 0.13 , OPTIC DIAMETERS 6.5 - 7 , ZONAL CURVATURES ARE

NE NE NE NE NE NE NE NE NE NE NE NE NE NE NE NE NE NE NE

FOR EDGE LIFT 0.13 , OPTIC DIAMETERS 7 - 7.5 , ZONAL CURVATURES ARE

42.55 49.15 57.75 69.5 86.3 NE NE NE NE NE NE NE NE NE NE NE NE NE NE

FOR EDGE LIFT 0.13 , OPTIC DIAMETERS 7.5 - 8 , ZONAL CURVATURES ARE

27 29.7 32.85 36.6 41.05 46.5 53.35 62.1 73.85 90.2 NE NE NE NE NE NE NE NE NE

FOR EDGE LIFT 0.13 , OPTIC DIAMETERS 8 - 8.5 , ZONAL CURVATURES ARE

20.1 21.65 23.4 25.3 27.5 30 32.9 36.25 40.15 44.85 50.5 57.55 66.45 78.15 94.2 NE NE NE NE

FOR EDGE LIFT 0.13 , OPTIC DIAMETERS 8.5 - 9 , ZONAL CURVATURES ARE

16.15 17.2 18.35 19.6 20.95 22.5 24.15 26 28.1 30.45 33.1 36.15 39.65 43.8 48.65 54.55 61.75 70.8 82.5

FOR EDGE LIFT 0.13 , OPTIC DIAMETERS 9 - 9.5 , ZONAL CURVATURES ARE

13.65 14.4 15.25 16.15 17.1 18.15 19.3 20.5 21.85 23.3 24.95 26.75 28.7 30.95 33.4 36.25 39.45 43.15 47.45

FOR EDGE LIFT 0.13 , OPTIC DIAMETERS 9.5 - 10 , ZONAL CURVATURES ARE

11.85 12.45 13.1 13.8 14.55 15.3 16.15 17.05 18.05 19.05 20.2 21.4 22.75 24.15 25.75 27.5 29.4 31.5 33.85

FOR EDGE LIFT 0.13 , OPTIC DIAMETERS 10 - 10.5 , ZONAL CURVATURES ARE

10.55 11.05 11.55 12.15 12.7 13.35 14 14.7 15.45 16.25 17.1 18 18.95 20 21.1 22.3 23.6 25.05 26.55

FOR EDGE LIFT 0.13 , OPTIC DIAMETERS 10.5 - 11 , ZONAL CURVATURES ARE

9.55 10 10.4 10.85 11.35 11.85 12.4 12.95 13.55 14.2 14.9 15.6 16.35 17.15 18 18.9 19.9 20.9 22.05

FOR EDGE LIFT 0.13 , OPTIC DIAMETERS 11 - 11.5 , ZONAL CURVATURES ARE

8.8 9.15 9.5 9.9 10.3 10.75 11.2 11.65 12.15 12.7 13.25 13.8 14.45 15.1 15.75 16.5 17.25 18.05 18.9

FOR EDGE LIFT 0.13 , OPTIC DIAMETERS 11.5 - 12 , ZONAL CURVATURES ARE

8.2 8.5 8.8 9.15 9.5 9.85 10.25 10.65 11.1 11.5 12 12.45 13 13.5 14.1 14.7 15.3 15.95 16.65

FOR EDGE LIFT 0.14 , OPTIC DIAMETERS 6 - 6.5 , ZONAL CURVATURES ARE

NE NE NE NE NE NE NE NE NE NE NE NE NE NE NE NE NE NE NE

FOR EDGE LIFT 0.14 , OPTIC DIAMETERS 6.5 - 7 , ZONAL CURVATURES ARE

NE NE NE NE NE NE NE NE NE NE NE NE NE NE NE NE NE NE NE

FOR EDGE LIFT 0.14 , OPTIC DIAMETERS 7 - 7.5 , ZONAL CURVATURES ARE

NE NE NE NE NE NE NE NE NE NE NE NE NE NE NE NE NE NE NE

FOR EDGE LIFT 0.14 , OPTIC DIAMETERS 7.5 - 8 , ZONAL CURVATURES ARE

37.15 42.5 49.35 58.35 NE NE NE NE NE NE NE NE NE NE NE NE NE NE NE

FOR EDGE LIFT 0.14 , OPTIC DIAMETERS 8 - 8.5 , ZONAL CURVATURES ARE

24.65 27.1 29.9 33.25 37.2 42 47.9 55.45 NE NE NE NE NE NE NE NE NE NE NE

FOR EDGE LIFT 0.14 , OPTIC DIAMETERS 8.5 - 9 , ZONAL CURVATURES ARE

18.65 20.15 21.75 23.55 25.6 27.95 30.65 33.75 37.45 41.8 47.05 53.55 61.8 NE NE NE NE NE NE

FOR EDGE LIFT 0.14 , OPTIC DIAMETERS 9 - 9.5 , ZONAL CURVATURES ARE

15.15 16.15 17.25 18.45 19.75 21.2 22.8 24.6 26.6 28.85 31.45 34.4 37.8 41.85 46.6 52.35 59.45 NE NE

FOR EDGE LIFT 0.14 , OPTIC DIAMETERS 9.5 - 10 , ZONAL CURVATURES ARE

12.8 13.55 14.35 15.25 16.2 17.2 18.3 19.5 20.8 22.25 23.85 25.6 27.6 29.8 32.25 35.1 38.3 42.05 46.45

FOR EDGE LIFT 0.14 , OPTIC DIAMETERS 10 - 10.5 , ZONAL CURVATURES ARE

11.2 11.75 12.4 13.05 13.8 14.55 15.35 16.25 17.2 18.25 19.35 20.55 21.9 23.35 24.9 26.65 28.6 30.75 33.15

FOR EDGE LIFT 0.14 , OPTIC DIAMETERS 10.5 - 11 , ZONAL CURVATURES ARE

10 10.45 10.95 11.5 12.05 12.7 13.3 14 14.75 15.55 16.4 17.3 18.25 19.3 20.4 21.65 22.95 24.4 25.95

FOR EDGE LIFT 0.14 , OPTIC DIAMETERS 11 - 11.5 , ZONAL CURVATURES ARE

9.05 9.45 9.9 10.3 10.8 11.3 11.8 12.35 12.95 13.6 14.25 14.95 15.7 16.55 17.4 18.3 19.3 20.35 21.45

FOR EDGE LIFT 0.14 , OPTIC DIAMETERS 11.5 - 12 , ZONAL CURVATURES ARE

8.35 8.7 9.05 9.4 9.8 10.25 10.65 11.15 11.6 12.15 12.7 13.25 13.85 14.5 15.2 15.95 16.7 17.5 18.4

```
FOR EDGE LIFT   0.15 ,   OPTIC DIAMETERS   6 - 6.5 ,   ZONAL CURVATURES ARE
NE NE NE NE NE NE NE NE NE NE NE NE NE NE NE NE NE NE NE

FOR EDGE LIFT   0.15 ,   OPTIC DIAMETERS   6.5 - 7 ,   ZONAL CURVATURES ARE
NE NE NE NE NE NE NE NE NE NE NE NE NE NE NE NE NE NE NE

FOR EDGE LIFT   0.15 ,   OPTIC DIAMETERS   7 - 7.5 ,   ZONAL CURVATURES ARE
NE NE NE NE NE NE NE NE NE NE NE NE NE NE NE NE NE NE NE

FOR EDGE LIFT   0.15 ,   OPTIC DIAMETERS   7.5 - 8 ,   ZONAL CURVATURES ARE
 59.8 NE NE NE NE NE NE NE NE NE NE NE NE NE NE NE NE NE NE

FOR EDGE LIFT   0.15 ,   OPTIC DIAMETERS   8 - 8.5 ,   ZONAL CURVATURES ARE
 32.1  36.4  41.75  48.65  57.75 NE NE NE NE NE NE NE NE NE NE NE NE NE NE

FOR EDGE LIFT   0.15 ,   OPTIC DIAMETERS   8.5 - 9 ,   ZONAL CURVATURES ARE
 22.2  24.35  26.8  29.7  33.1  37.2  42.2  48.45  56.5 NE NE NE NE NE NE NE NE NE NE

FOR EDGE LIFT   0.15 ,   OPTIC DIAMETERS   9 - 9.5 ,   ZONAL CURVATURES ARE
 17.1  18.45  19.95  21.6  23.5  25.6  28.05  30.85  34.2  38.1  42.8  48.55  55.8 NE NE NE NE NE NE

FOR EDGE LIFT   0.15 ,   OPTIC DIAMETERS   9.5 - 10 ,   ZONAL CURVATURES ARE
 14  14.95  15.95  17.1  18.3  19.7  21.2  22.85  24.75  26.85  29.3  32.05  35.25  39  43.5  48.85  55.45  63.75 NE

FOR EDGE LIFT   0.15 ,   OPTIC DIAMETERS   10 - 10.5 ,   ZONAL CURVATURES ARE
 11.95  12.65  13.4  14.2  15.1  16.05  17.15  18.25  19.55  20.9  22.45  24.15  26  28.15  30.55  33.25  36.4  40  44.25

FOR EDGE LIFT   0.15 ,   OPTIC DIAMETERS   10.5 - 11 ,   ZONAL CURVATURES ARE
 10.45  11  11.6  12.25  12.9  13.65  14.45  15.3  16.2  17.2  18.3  19.45  20.75  22.15  23.7  25.4  27.3  29.4  31.8

FOR EDGE LIFT   0.15 ,   OPTIC DIAMETERS   11 - 11.5 ,   ZONAL CURVATURES ARE
 9.35  9.8  10.3  10.8  11.35  11.95  12.55  13.2  13.95  14.7  15.5  16.4  17.35  18.35  19.45  20.65  21.95  23.4  24.95

FOR EDGE LIFT   0.15 ,   OPTIC DIAMETERS   11.5 - 12 ,   ZONAL CURVATURES ARE
 8.55  8.9  9.3  9.75  10.2  10.65  11.15  11.7  12.25  12.85  13.5  14.2  14.95  15.75  16.6  17.5  18.45  19.5  20.65
```

TABLE V Back Peripheral Optic Radii (Zonal Curvatures) for the following:
BCOR 7.0 to 8.8 in 0.1 steps
Zone Width 0.3 Zone Inner Diameters 7.0 to 10.4 in 0.2 steps
Axial Edge Lift Components 0.01 to 0.15 in 0.01 steps

```
FOR EDGE LIFT   0.01 ,   OPTIC DIAMETERS   7  -  7.6 ,    ZONAL CURVATURES ARE
 7.3  7.4  7.5  7.65  7.75  7.85  8  8.1  8.2  8.35  8.45  8.55  8.7  8.8  8.9  9.05  9.15  9.25  9.4

FOR EDGE LIFT   0.01 ,   OPTIC DIAMETERS   7.2  -  7.8 ,    ZONAL CURVATURES ARE
 7.3  7.4  7.5  7.6  7.75  7.85  7.95  8.1  8.2  8.3  8.4  8.55  8.65  8.75  8.9  9  9.1  9.25  9.35

FOR EDGE LIFT   0.01 ,   OPTIC DIAMETERS   7.4  -  8 ,    ZONAL CURVATURES ARE
 7.25  7.35  7.5  7.6  7.7  7.85  7.95  8.05  8.15  8.3  8.4  8.5  8.65  8.75  8.85  9  9.1  9.2  9.35

FOR EDGE LIFT   0.01 ,   OPTIC DIAMETERS   7.6  -  8.2 ,    ZONAL CURVATURES ARE
 7.25  7.35  7.45  7.6  7.7  7.8  7.9  8.05  8.15  8.25  8.4  8.5  8.6  8.7  8.85  8.95  9.05  9.2  9.3

FOR EDGE LIFT   0.01 ,   OPTIC DIAMETERS   7.8  -  8.4 ,    ZONAL CURVATURES ARE
 7.25  7.35  7.45  7.55  7.7  7.8  7.9  8  8.15  8.25  8.35  8.45  8.6  8.7  8.8  8.95  9.05  9.15  9.3

FOR EDGE LIFT   0.01 ,   OPTIC DIAMETERS   8.  -  8.6 ,    ZONAL CURVATURES ARE
 7.2  7.35  7.45  7.55  7.65  7.8  7.9  8  8.1  8.25  8.35  8.45  8.55  8.7  8.8  8.9  9.05  9.15  9.25

FOR EDGE LIFT   0.01 ,   OPTIC DIAMETERS   8.2  -  8.8 ,    ZONAL CURVATURES ARE
 7.2  7.3  7.45  7.55  7.65  7.75  7.85  8  8.1  8.2  8.3  8.45  8.55  8.65  8.8  8.9  9  9.1  9.25

FOR EDGE LIFT   0.01 ,   OPTIC DIAMETERS   8.4  -  9 ,    ZONAL CURVATURES ARE
 7.2  7.3  7.4  7.5  7.65  7.75  7.85  7.95  8.1  8.2  8.3  8.4  8.55  8.65  8.75  8.85  9  9.1  9.2
```

FOR EDGE LIFT 0.01 , OPTIC DIAMETERS 8.6 - 9.2 , ZONAL CURVATURES ARE

7.2 7.3 7.4 7.5 7.6 7.75 7.85 7.95 8.05 8.2 8.3 8.4 8.5 8.65 8.75 8.85 8.95 9.1 9.2

FOR EDGE LIFT 0.01 , OPTIC DIAMETERS 8.8 - 9.4 , ZONAL CURVATURES ARE

7.15 7.3 7.4 7.5 7.6 7.7 7.85 7.95 8.05 8.15 3.3 8.4 8.5 8.6 8.75 8.85 8.95 9.05 9.2

FOR EDGE LIFT 0.01 , OPTIC DIAMETERS 9. - 9.6 , ZONAL CURVATURES ARE

7.15 7.25 7.35 7.5 7.6 7.7 7.8 7.95 8.05 8.15 8.25 8.35 8.5 8.6 8.7 8.8 8.95 9.05 9.15

FOR EDGE LIFT 0.01 , OPTIC DIAMETERS 9.2 - 9.8 , ZONAL CURVATURES ARE

7.15 7.25 7.35 7.45 7.6 7.7 7.8 7.9 8 8.15 8.25 8.35 8.45 8.6 8.7 8.8 8.9 9.05 9.15

FOR EDGE LIFT 0.01 , OPTIC DIAMETERS 9.4 - 10. , ZONAL CURVATURES ARE

7.15 7.25 7.35 7.45 7.55 7.7 7.8 7.9 8 8.1 8.25 8.35 8.45 8.55 8.7 8.8 8.9 9 9.15

FOR EDGE LIFT 0.01 , OPTIC DIAMETERS 9.6 - 10.2 , ZONAL CURVATURES ARE

7.1 7.25 7.35 7.45 7.55 7.65 7.8 7.9 8 8.1 8.2 8.35 8.45 8.55 8.65 8.8 8.9 9 9.1

FOR EDGE LIFT 0.01 , OPTIC DIAMETERS 9.8 - 10.4 , ZONAL CURVATURES ARE

7.1 7.2 7.35 7.45 7.55 7.65 7.75 7.9 8 8.1 8.2 8.3 8.45 8.55 8.65 8.75 8.85 9 9.1

FOR EDGE LIFT 0.01 , OPTIC DIAMETERS 10. - 10.6 , ZONAL CURVATURES ARE

7.1 7.2 7.3 7.45 7.55 7.65 7.75 7.85 7.95 8.1 8.2 8.3 8.4 8.55 8.65 8.75 8.85 8.95 9.1

FOR EDGE LIFT 0.01 , OPTIC DIAMETERS 10.2 - 10.8 , ZONAL CURVATURES ARE

7.1 7.2 7.3 7.4 7.55 7.65 7.75 7.85 7.95 8.05 8.2 8.3 8.4 8.5 8.6 8.75 8.85 8.95 9.05

FOR EDGE LIFT 0.01 , OPTIC DIAMETERS 10.4 - 11. , ZONAL CURVATURES ARE

7.1 7.2 7.3 7.4 7.5 7.65 7.75 7.85 7.95 8.05 8.15 8.3 8.4 8.5 8.6 8.7 8.85 8.95 9.05

```
FOR EDGE LIFT   0.02 ,   OPTIC DIAMETERS   7 - 7.6 ,   ZONAL CURVATURES ARE
 7.65  7.75  7.9  8  8.15  8.3  8.4  8.55  8.7  8.8  8.95  9.1  9.25  9.35  9.5  9.65  9.8  9.9  10.05

FOR EDGE LIFT   0.02 ,   OPTIC DIAMETERS   7.2 - 7.8 ,   ZONAL CURVATURES ARE
 7.6  7.7  7.85  8  8.1  8.25  8.4  8.5  8.65  8.75  8.9  9.05  9.2  9.3  9.45  9.6  9.75  9.85  10

FOR EDGE LIFT   0.02 ,   OPTIC DIAMETERS   7.4 - 8 ,   ZONAL CURVATURES ARE
 7.55  7.7  7.8  7.95  8.05  8.2  8.35  8.45  8.6  8.75  8.85  9  9.15  9.25  9.4  9.55  9.65  9.8  9.95

FOR EDGE LIFT   0.02 ,   OPTIC DIAMETERS   7.6 - 8.2 ,   ZONAL CURVATURES ARE
 7.5  7.65  7.8  7.9  8.05  8.15  8.3  8.4  8.55  8.7  8.8  8.95  9.1  9.2  9.35  9.5  9.6  9.75  9.9

FOR EDGE LIFT   0.02 ,   OPTIC DIAMETERS   7.8 - 8.4 ,   ZONAL CURVATURES ARE
 7.5  7.6  7.75  7.85  8  8.1  8.25  8.4  8.5  8.65  8.75  8.9  9.05  9.15  9.3  9.45  9.55  9.7  9.85

FOR EDGE LIFT   0.02 ,   OPTIC DIAMETERS   8. - 8.6 ,   ZONAL CURVATURES ARE
 7.45  7.6  7.7  7.85  7.95  8.1  8.2  8.35  8.45  8.6  8.75  8.85  9  9.1  9.25  9.4  9.5  9.65  9.8

FOR EDGE LIFT   0.02 ,   OPTIC DIAMETERS   8.2 - 8.8 ,   ZONAL CURVATURES ARE
 7.45  7.55  7.7  7.8  7.95  8.05  8.2  8.3  8.45  8.55  8.7  8.8  8.95  9.1  9.2  9.35  9.5  9.6  9.75

FOR EDGE LIFT   0.02 ,   OPTIC DIAMETERS   8.4 - 9 ,   ZONAL CURVATURES ARE
 7.4  7.5  7.65  7.75  7.9  8  8.15  8.25  8.4  8.55  8.65  8.8  8.9  9.05  9.15  9.3  9.45  9.55  9.7

FOR EDGE LIFT   0.02 ,   OPTIC DIAMETERS   8.6 - 9.2 ,   ZONAL CURVATURES ARE
 7.35  7.5  7.6  7.75  7.85  8  8.1  8.25  8.35  8.5  8.6  8.75  8.9  9  9.15  9.25  9.4  9.5  9.65
```

```
FOR EDGE LIFT   0.02 ,   OPTIC DIAMETERS   8.8  -  9.4 ,    ZONAL CURVATURES ARE
 7.35  7.45  7.6  7.7  7.85  7.95  8.1  8.2  8.35  8.45  8.5  8.7  8.85  8.95  9.1  9.2  9.35  9.5  9.6

FOR EDGE LIFT   0.02 ,   OPTIC DIAMETERS   9.  -  9.6 ,    ZONAL CURVATURES ARE
 7.3  7.45  7.55  7.7  7.8  7.95  8.05  8.2  8.3  8.45  8.55  8.7  8.8  8.95  9.05  9.2  9.3  9.45  9.55

FOR EDGE LIFT   0.02 ,   OPTIC DIAMETERS   9.2  -  9.8 ,    ZONAL CURVATURES ARE
 7.3  7.4  7.55  7.65  7.8  7.9  8.05  8.15  8.25  8.4  8.5  8.65  8.75  8.9  9  9.15  9.3  9.4  9.55

FOR EDGE LIFT   0.02 ,   OPTIC DIAMETERS   9.4  -  10. ,    ZONAL CURVATURES ARE
 7.3  7.4  7.5  7.65  7.75  7.9  8  8.1  8.25  8.35  8.5  8.6  8.75  8.85  9  9.1  9.25  9.35  9.5

FOR EDGE LIFT   0.02 ,   OPTIC DIAMETERS   9.6  -  10.2 ,    ZONAL CURVATURES ARE
 7.25  7.35  7.5  7.6  7.75  7.85  7.95  8.1  8.2  8.35  8.45  8.6  8.7  8.85  8.95  9.1  9.2  9.35  9.45

FOR EDGE LIFT   0.02 ,   OPTIC DIAMETERS   9.8  -  10.4 ,    ZONAL CURVATURES ARE
 7.25  7.35  7.45  7.6  7.7  7.85  7.95  8.05  8.2  8.3  8.45  8.55  8.7  8.8  8.95  9.05  9.2  9.3  9.45

FOR EDGE LIFT   0.02 ,   OPTIC DIAMETERS   10.  -  10.6 ,    ZONAL CURVATURES ARE
 7.2  7.35  7.45  7.55  7.7  7.8  7.95  8.05  8.15  8.3  8.4  8.55  8.65  8.8  8.9  9  9.15  9.25  9.4

FOR EDGE LIFT   0.02 ,   OPTIC DIAMETERS   10.2  -  10.8 ,    ZONAL CURVATURES ARE
 7.2  7.3  7.45  7.55  7.65  7.8  7.9  8  8.15  8.25  8.4  8.5  8.65  8.75  8.85  9  9.1  9.25  9.35

FOR EDGE LIFT   0.02 ,   OPTIC DIAMETERS   10.4  -  11. ,    ZONAL CURVATURES ARE
 7.2  7.3  7.4  7.55  7.65  7.75  7.9  8  8.1  8.25  8.35  8.5  8.6  8.7  8.85  8.95  9.1  9.2  9.35
```

```
FOR EDGE LIFT   0.03 ,   OPTIC DIAMETERS   7 - 7.6 ,    ZONAL CURVATURES ARE
 8  8.15  8.3  8.45  8.6  8.8  8.95  9.1  9.25  9.4  9.55  9.75  9.9  10.05  10.2  10.4  10.55  10.7  10.9

FOR EDGE LIFT   0.03 ,   OPTIC DIAMETERS   7.2 - 7.8 ,    ZONAL CURVATURES ARE
 7.95  8.1  8.25  8.4  8.55  8.7  8.85  9  9.15  9.3  9.5  9.65  9.8  9.95  10.1  10.3  10.45  10.6  10.8

FOR EDGE LIFT   0.03 ,   OPTIC DIAMETERS   7.4 - 8 ,    ZONAL CURVATURES ARE
 7.9  8.05  8.2  8.35  8.5  8.65  8.8  8.95  9.1  9.25  9.4  9.55  9.7  9.85  10.05  10.2  10.35  10.5  10.7

FOR EDGE LIFT   0.03 ,   OPTIC DIAMETERS   7.6 - 8.2 ,    ZONAL CURVATURES ARE
 7.85  8  8.15  8.25  8.4  8.55  8.7  8.85  9  9.15  9.3  9.45  9.65  9.8  9.95  10.1  10.25  10.4  10.6

FOR EDGE LIFT   0.03 ,   OPTIC DIAMETERS   7.8 - 8.4 ,    ZONAL CURVATURES ARE
 7.8  7.9  8.05  8.2  8.35  8.5  8.65  8.8  8.95  9.1  9.25  9.4  9.55  9.7  9.85  10  10.15  10.35  10.5

FOR EDGE LIFT   0.03 ,   OPTIC DIAMETERS   8. - 8.6 ,    ZONAL CURVATURES ARE
 7.75  7.85  8  8.15  8.3  8.45  8.6  8.75  8.9  9.05  9.2  9.35  9.5  9.65  9.8  9.95  10.1  10.25  10.4

FOR EDGE LIFT   0.03 ,   OPTIC DIAMETERS   8.2 - 8.8 ,    ZONAL CURVATURES ARE
 7.7  7.8  7.95  8.1  8.25  8.4  8.55  8.65  8.8  8.95  9.1  9.25  9.4  9.55  9.7  9.85  10  10.15  10.35

FOR EDGE LIFT   0.03 ,   OPTIC DIAMETERS   8.4 - 9 ,    ZONAL CURVATURES ARE
 7.65  7.75  7.9  8.05  8.2  8.35  8.45  8.6  8.75  8.9  9.05  9.2  9.35  9.5  9.65  9.8  9.95  10.1  10.25

FOR EDGE LIFT   0.03 ,   OPTIC DIAMETERS   8.6 - 9.2 ,    ZONAL CURVATURES ARE
 7.6  7.75  7.85  8  8.15  8.3  8.4  8.55  8.7  8.85  9  9.15  9.3  9.45  9.6  9.75  9.9  10.05  10.2
```

```
FOR EDGE LIFT   0.03 ,   OPTIC DIAMETERS   8.8  -  9.4 ,    ZONAL CURVATURES ARE
 7.55  7.7  7.8  7.95  8.1  8.25  8.35  8.5  8.65  8.8  8.95  9.1  9.2  9.35  9.5  9.65  9.8  9.95  10.1

FOR EDGE LIFT   0.03 ,   OPTIC DIAMETERS   9.  -  9.6 ,    ZONAL CURVATURES ARE
 7.5  7.65  7.8  7.9  8.05  8.2  8.3  8.45  8.6  8.75  8.9  9  9.15  9.3  9.45  9.6  9.75  9.9  10.05

FOR EDGE LIFT   0.03 ,   OPTIC DIAMETERS   9.2  -  9.8 ,    ZONAL CURVATURES ARE
 7.45  7.6  7.75  7.85  8  8.15  8.3  8.4  8.55  8.7  8.85  8.95  9.1  9.25  9.4  9.55  9.7  9.85  10

FOR EDGE LIFT   0.03 ,   OPTIC DIAMETERS   9.4  -  10. ,    ZONAL CURVATURES ARE
 7.45  7.55  7.7  7.85  7.95  8.1  8.25  8.35  8.5  8.65  8.8  8.9  9.05  9.2  9.35  9.5  9.65  9.75  9.9

FOR EDGE LIFT   0.03 ,   OPTIC DIAMETERS   9.6  -  10.2 ,    ZONAL CURVATURES ARE
 7.4  7.55  7.65  7.8  7.9  8.05  8.2  8.35  8.45  8.6  8.75  8.85  9  9.15  9.3  9.45  9.55  9.7  9.85

FOR EDGE LIFT   0.03 ,   OPTIC DIAMETERS   9.8  -  10.4 ,    ZONAL CURVATURES ARE
 7.35  7.5  7.6  7.75  7.9  8  8.15  8.3  8.4  8.55  8.7  8.85  8.95  9.1  9.25  9.4  9.5  9.65  9.8

FOR EDGE LIFT   0.03 ,   OPTIC DIAMETERS   10.  -  10.6 ,    ZONAL CURVATURES ARE
 7.35  7.45  7.6  7.7  7.85  8  8.1  8.25  8.4  8.5  8.65  8.8  8.9  9.05  9.2  9.35  9.45  9.6  9.75

FOR EDGE LIFT   0.03 ,   OPTIC DIAMETERS   10.2  -  10.8 ,    ZONAL CURVATURES ARE
 7.3  7.45  7.55  7.7  7.8  7.95  8.1  8.2  8.35  8.45  8.6  8.75  8.9  9  9.15  9.3  9.4  9.55  9.7

FOR EDGE LIFT   0.03 ,   OPTIC DIAMETERS   10.4  -  11. ,    ZONAL CURVATURES ARE
 7.25  7.4  7.55  7.65  7.8  7.9  8.05  8.15  8.3  8.45  8.55  8.7  8.85  8.95  9.1  9.25  9.4  9.5  9.65
```

```
FOR EDGE LIFT   0.04 ,   OPTIC DIAMETERS   7 - 7.6 ,   ZONAL CURVATURES ARE
 8.45  8.65  8.8  9  9.15  9.35  9.55  9.7  9.9  10.1  10.3  10.5  10.7  10.85  11.05  11.25  11.5  11.7  11.9

FOR EDGE LIFT   0.04 ,   OPTIC DIAMETERS   7.2 - 7.8 ,   ZONAL CURVATURES ARE
 8.35  8.55  8.7  8.9  9.05  9.25  9.4  9.6  9.8  9.95  10.15  10.35  10.55  10.75  10.9  11.1  11.3  11.5  11.7

FOR EDGE LIFT   0.04 ,   OPTIC DIAMETERS   7.4 - 8 ,   ZONAL CURVATURES ARE
 8.3  8.45  8.6  8.8  8.95  9.15  9.3  9.5  9.65  9.85  10.05  10.2  10.4  10.6  10.8  10.95  11.15  11.35  11.55

FOR EDGE LIFT   0.04 ,   OPTIC DIAMETERS   7.6 - 8.2 ,   ZONAL CURVATURES ARE
 8.2  8.35  8.5  8.7  8.85  9.05  9.2  9.4  9.55  9.75  9.9  10.1  10.25  10.45  10.65  10.85  11  11.2  11.4

FOR EDGE LIFT   0.04 ,   OPTIC DIAMETERS   7.8 - 8.4 ,   ZONAL CURVATURES ARE
 8.1  8.25  8.45  8.6  8.75  8.95  9.1  9.3  9.45  9.6  9.8  10  10.15  10.35  10.5  10.7  10.9  11.1  11.25

FOR EDGE LIFT   0.04 ,   OPTIC DIAMETERS   8. - 8.6 ,   ZONAL CURVATURES ARE
 8.05  8.2  8.35  8.5  8.7  8.85  9  9.2  9.35  9.5  9.7  9.85  10.05  10.2  10.4  10.6  10.75  10.95  11.15

FOR EDGE LIFT   0.04 ,   OPTIC DIAMETERS   8.2 - 8.8 ,   ZONAL CURVATURES ARE
 7.95  8.1  8.3  8.45  8.6  8.75  8.95  9.1  9.25  9.45  9.6  9.75  9.95  10.1  10.3  10.45  10.65  10.85  11

FOR EDGE LIFT   0.04 ,   OPTIC DIAMETERS   8.4 - 9 ,   ZONAL CURVATURES ARE
 7.9  8.05  8.2  8.35  8.5  8.7  8.85  9  9.15  9.35  9.5  9.65  9.85  10  10.2  10.35  10.55  10.7  10.9

FOR EDGE LIFT   0.04 ,   OPTIC DIAMETERS   8.6 - 9.2 ,   ZONAL CURVATURES ARE
 7.85  8  8.15  8.3  8.45  8.6  8.75  8.95  9.1  9.25  9.4  9.6  9.75  9.9  10.1  10.25  10.45  10.6  10.8
```

```
FOR EDGE LIFT   0.04 ,   OPTIC DIAMETERS   8.8  -  9.4 ,   ZONAL CURVATURES ARE
 7.75  7.9  8.05  8.25  8.4  8.55  8.7  8.85  9  9.15  9.35  9.5  9.65  9.85  10  10.15  10.35  10.5  10.7

FOR EDGE LIFT   0.04 ,   OPTIC DIAMETERS   9.  -  9.6 ,   ZONAL CURVATURES ARE
 7.7  7.85  8  8.15  8.3  8.45  8.6  8.8  8.95  9.1  9.25  9.4  9.6  9.75  9.9  10.05  10.25  10.4  10.6

FOR EDGE LIFT   0.04 ,   OPTIC DIAMETERS   9.2  -  9.8 ,   ZONAL CURVATURES ARE
 7.65  7.8  7.95  8.1  8.25  8.4  8.55  8.7  8.85  9  9.2  9.35  9.5  9.65  9.8  10  10.15  10.3  10.5

FOR EDGE LIFT   0.04 ,   OPTIC DIAMETERS   9.4  -  10. ,   ZONAL CURVATURES ARE
 7.6  7.75  7.9  8.05  8.2  8.35  8.5  8.65  8.8  8.95  9.1  9.25  9.4  9.6  9.75  9.9  10.05  10.25  10.4

FOR EDGE LIFT   0.04 ,   OPTIC DIAMETERS   9.6  -  10.2 ,   ZONAL CURVATURES ARE
 7.55  7.7  7.85  8  8.15  8.3  8.45  8.6  8.75  8.9  9.05  9.2  9.35  9.5  9.65  9.85  10  10.15  10.3

FOR EDGE LIFT   0.04 ,   OPTIC DIAMETERS   9.8  -  10.4 ,   ZONAL CURVATURES ARE
 7.5  7.65  7.8  7.95  8.1  8.25  8.35  8.5  8.65  8.8  8.95  9.15  9.3  9.45  9.6  9.75  9.9  10.05  10.25

FOR EDGE LIFT   0.04 ,   OPTIC DIAMETERS   10.  -  10.6 ,   ZONAL CURVATURES ARE
 7.45  7.6  7.75  7.9  8.05  8.15  8.3  8.45  3.6  8.75  8.9  9.05  9.2  9.35  9.5  9.7  9.85  10  10.15

FOR EDGE LIFT   0.04 ,   OPTIC DIAMETERS   10.2  -  10.8 ,   ZONAL CURVATURES ARE
 7.4  7.55  7.7  7.85  8  3.1  8.25  8.4  8.55  8.7  8.85  9  9.15  9.3  9.45  9.6  9.75  9.9  10.1

FOR EDGE LIFT   0.04 ,   OPTIC DIAMETERS   10.4  -  11. ,   ZONAL CURVATURES ARE
 7.4  7.5  7.65  7.8  7.95  8.05  8.2  8.35  8.5  8.65  8.8  8.95  9.1  9.25  9.4  9.55  9.7  9.85  10
```

```
FOR EDGE LIFT   0.05 ,   OPTIC DIAMETERS   7 - 7.6 ,   ZONAL CURVATURES ARE
 9  9.2  9.4  9.6  9.8  10.05  10.25  10.45  10.7  10.95  11.15  11.4  11.65  11.85  12.1  12.35  12.6  12.9  13.15

FOR EDGE LIFT   0.05 ,   OPTIC DIAMETERS   7.2 - 7.8 ,   ZONAL CURVATURES ARE
 8.85  9.05  9.25  9.45  9.65  9.85  10.1  10.3  10.5  10.75  10.95  11.2  11.4  11.65  11.9  12.15  12.4  12.6  12.9

FOR EDGE LIFT   0.05 ,   OPTIC DIAMETERS   7.4 - 8 ,   ZONAL CURVATURES ARE
 8.7  8.9  9.1  9.3  9.5  9.7  9.9  10.15  10.35  10.55  10.8  11  11.2  11.45  11.7  11.9  12.15  12.4  12.65

FOR EDGE LIFT   0.05 ,   OPTIC DIAMETERS   7.6 - 8.2 ,   ZONAL CURVATURES ARE
 8.6  8.8  9  9.2  9.35  9.55  9.75  10  10.2  10.4  10.6  10.8  11.05  11.25  11.5  11.7  11.95  12.15  12.4

FOR EDGE LIFT   0.05 ,   OPTIC DIAMETERS   7.8 - 8.4 ,   ZONAL CURVATURES ARE
 8.5  8.65  8.85  9.05  9.25  9.45  9.65  9.85  10.05  10.25  10.45  10.65  10.85  11.1  11.3  11.5  11.75  11.95  12.2

FOR EDGE LIFT   0.05 ,   OPTIC DIAMETERS   8. - 8.6 ,   ZONAL CURVATURES ARE
 8.4  8.55  8.75  8.95  9.1  9.3  9.5  9.7  9.9  10.1  10.3  10.5  10.7  10.9  11.15  11.35  11.55  11.8  12

FOR EDGE LIFT   0.05 ,   OPTIC DIAMETERS   8.2 - 8.8 ,   ZONAL CURVATURES ARE
 8.3  8.45  8.65  8.8  9  9.2  9.4  9.55  9.75  9.95  10.15  10.35  10.55  10.75  10.95  11.2  11.4  11.6  11.85

FOR EDGE LIFT   0.05 ,   OPTIC DIAMETERS   8.4 - 9 ,   ZONAL CURVATURES ARE
 8.2  8.35  8.55  8.7  8.9  9.1  9.25  9.45  9.65  9.85  10.05  10.2  10.4  10.6  10.85  11.05  11.25  11.45  11.65

FOR EDGE LIFT   0.05 ,   OPTIC DIAMETERS   8.6 - 9.2 ,   ZONAL CURVATURES ARE
 8.1  8.25  8.45  8.6  8.8  9  9.15  9.35  9.55  9.7  9.9  10.1  10.3  10.5  10.7  10.9  11.1  11.3  11.5
```

```
FOR EDGE LIFT   0.05 ,   OPTIC DIAMETERS   8.8  -  9.4 ,    ZONAL CURVATURES ARE
 8  8.2  8.35  8.55  8.7  8.9  9.05  9.25  9.4  9.6  9.8  10  10.15  10.35  10.55  10.75  10.95  11.15  11.35

FOR EDGE LIFT   0.05 ,   OPTIC DIAMETERS   9.  -  9.6 ,    ZONAL CURVATURES ARE
 7.95  8.1  8.25  8.45  8.6  8.8  8.95  9.15  9.3  9.5  9.7  9.85  10.05  10.25  10.45  10.6  10.8  11  11.2

FOR EDGE LIFT   0.05 ,   OPTIC DIAMETERS   9.2  -  9.8 ,    ZONAL CURVATURES ARE
 7.85  8.05  8.2  8.35  8.55  8.7  8.85  9.05  9.2  9.4  9.55  9.75  9.95  10.1  10.3  10.5  10.7  10.9  11.1

FOR EDGE LIFT   0.05 ,   OPTIC DIAMETERS   9.4  -  10. ,    ZONAL CURVATURES ARE
 7.8  7.95  8.1  8.3  8.45  8.6  8.8  8.95  9.1  9.3  9.5  9.65  9.85  10  10.2  10.4  10.55  10.75  10.95

FOR EDGE LIFT   0.05 ,   OPTIC DIAMETERS   9.6  -  10.2 ,    ZONAL CURVATURES ARE
 7.75  7.9  8.05  8.2  8.35  8.55  8.7  8.85  9.05  9.2  9.4  9.55  9.75  9.9  10.1  10.25  10.45  10.65  10.85

FOR EDGE LIFT   0.05 ,   OPTIC DIAMETERS   9.8  -  10.4 ,    ZONAL CURVATURES ARE
 7.65  7.8  8  8.15  8.3  8.45  8.6  8.8  8.95  9.1  9.3  9.45  9.65  9.8  10  10.15  10.35  10.55  10.7

FOR EDGE LIFT   0.05 ,   OPTIC DIAMETERS   10.  -  10.6 ,    ZONAL CURVATURES ARE
 7.6  7.75  7.9  8.05  8.25  8.4  8.55  8.7  8.85  9.05  9.2  9.4  9.55  9.7  9.9  10.05  10.25  10.45  10.6

FOR EDGE LIFT   0.05 ,   OPTIC DIAMETERS   10.2  -  10.8 ,    ZONAL CURVATURES ARE
 7.55  7.7  7.85  8  8.15  8.3  8.5  8.65  8.8  8.95  9.15  9.3  9.45  9.65  9.8  10  10.15  10.35  10.5

FOR EDGE LIFT   0.05 ,   OPTIC DIAMETERS   10.4  -  11. ,    ZONAL CURVATURES ARE
 7.5  7.65  7.8  7.95  8.1  8.25  8.4  8.55  8.75  8.9  9.05  9.2  9.4  9.55  9.7  9.9  10.05  10.25  10.4
```

```
FOR EDGE LIFT   6.00000E-2 ,   OPTIC DIAMETERS   7  -  7.6 ,   ZONAL CURVATURES ARE
 9.6  9.85  10.1  10.35  10.6  10.85  11.1  11.4  11.65  11.95  12.2  12.5  12.8  13.1  13.4  13.75  14.05  14.4  14.7

FOR EDGE LIFT   6.00000E-2 ,   OPTIC DIAMETERS   7.2  -  7.8 ,   ZONAL CURVATURES ARE
 9.4  9.65  9.9  10.1  10.35  10.6  10.85  11.15  11.4  11.65  11.95  12.2  12.5  12.8  13.1  13.4  13.7  14  14.35

FOR EDGE LIFT   6.00000E-2 ,   OPTIC DIAMETERS   7.4  -  8 ,   ZONAL CURVATURES ARE
 9.25  9.45  9.7  9.9  10.15  10.4  10.65  10.9  11.15  11.4  11.7  11.95  12.2  12.5  12.8  13.05  13.35  13.65  13.95

FOR EDGE LIFT   6.00000E-2 ,   OPTIC DIAMETERS   7.6  -  8.2 ,   ZONAL CURVATURES ARE
 9.05  9.3  9.5  9.75  9.95  10.2  10.45  10.7  10.95  11.2  11.45  11.7  11.95  12.25  12.5  12.8  13.05  13.35  13.65

FOR EDGE LIFT   6.00000E-2 ,   OPTIC DIAMETERS   7.8  -  8.4 ,   ZONAL CURVATURES ARE
 8.9  9.15  9.35  9.55  9.8  10  10.25  10.5  10.75  10.95  11.2  11.45  11.7  12  12.25  12.5  12.8  13.05  13.35

FOR EDGE LIFT   6.00000E-2 ,   OPTIC DIAMETERS   8.  -  8.6 ,   ZONAL CURVATURES ARE
 8.8  9  9.2  9.4  9.65  9.85  10.1  10.3  10.55  10.75  11  11.25  11.5  11.75  12  12.25  12.55  12.8  13.05

FOR EDGE LIFT   6.00000E-2 ,   OPTIC DIAMETERS   8.2  -  8.8 ,   ZONAL CURVATURES ARE
 8.65  8.85  9.05  9.25  9.5  9.7  9.9  10.15  10.35  10.6  10.8  11.05  11.3  11.55  11.8  12.05  12.3  12.55  12.8

FOR EDGE LIFT   6.00000E-2 ,   OPTIC DIAMETERS   8.4  -  9 ,   ZONAL CURVATURES ARE
 8.5  8.7  8.9  9.15  9.35  9.55  9.75  9.95  10.2  10.4  10.65  10.85  11.1  11.35  11.6  11.8  12.05  12.3  12.55

FOR EDGE LIFT   6.00000E-2 ,   OPTIC DIAMETERS   8.6  -  9.2 ,   ZONAL CURVATURES ARE
 8.4  8.6  8.8  9  9.2  9.4  9.6  9.8  10.05  10.25  10.45  10.7  10.9  11.15  11.4  11.6  11.85  12.1  12.35
```

```
FOR EDGE LIFT   6.00000E-2 ,   OPTIC DIAMETERS   8.8  -  9.4 ,    ZONAL CURVATURES ARE
 8.3  8.5  8.7  8.85  9.05  9.25  9.45  9.7  9.9  10.1  10.3  10.55  10.75  10.95  11.2  11.45  11.65  11.9  12.15

FOR EDGE LIFT   6.00000E-2 ,   OPTIC DIAMETERS   9.  -  9.6 ,    ZONAL CURVATURES ARE
 8.2  8.4  8.55  8.75  8.95  9.15  9.35  9.55  9.75  9.95  10.15  10.4  10.6  10.8  11.05  11.25  11.5  11.7  11.95

FOR EDGE LIFT   6.00000E-2 ,   OPTIC DIAMETERS   9.2  -  9.8 ,    ZONAL CURVATURES ARE
 8.1  8.3  8.45  8.65  8.85  9.05  9.2  9.4  9.6  9.8  10  10.25  10.45  10.65  10.85  11.1  11.3  11.55  11.75

FOR EDGE LIFT   6.00000E-2 ,   OPTIC DIAMETERS   9.4  -  10. ,    ZONAL CURVATURES ARE
 8  8.2  8.35  8.55  8.75  8.9  9.1  9.3  9.5  9.7  9.9  10.1  10.3  10.5  10.7  10.95  11.15  11.35  11.6

FOR EDGE LIFT   6.00000E-2 ,   OPTIC DIAMETERS   9.6  -  10.2 ,    ZONAL CURVATURES ARE
 7.9  8.1  8.25  8.45  8.65  8.8  9  9.2  9.4  9.55  9.75  9.95  10.15  10.35  10.6  10.8  11  11.2  11.45

FOR EDGE LIFT   6.00000E-2 ,   OPTIC DIAMETERS   9.8  -  10.4 ,    ZONAL CURVATURES ARE
 7.85  8  8.2  8.35  8.55  8.7  8.9  9.1  9.25  9.45  9.65  9.85  10.05  10.25  10.45  10.65  10.85  11.05  11.3

FOR EDGE LIFT   6.00000E-2 ,   OPTIC DIAMETERS   10.  -  10.6 ,    ZONAL CURVATURES ARE
 7.75  7.95  8.1  8.25  8.45  8.6  8.8  9  9.15  9.35  9.55  9.75  9.9  10.1  10.3  10.5  10.7  10.9  11.15

FOR EDGE LIFT   6.00000E-2 ,   OPTIC DIAMETERS   10.2  -  10.8 ,    ZONAL CURVATURES ARE
 7.7  7.85  8  8.2  8.35  8.55  8.7  8.9  9.05  9.25  9.45  9.6  9.8  10  10.2  10.4  10.6  10.8  11

FOR EDGE LIFT   6.00000E-2 ,   OPTIC DIAMETERS   10.4  -  11. ,    ZONAL CURVATURES ARE
 7.6  7.8  7.95  8.1  8.3  8.45  8.6  8.8  8.95  9.15  9.35  9.5  9.7  9.9  10.1  10.25  10.45  10.65  10.85
```

FOR EDGE LIFT 0.07 , OPTIC DIAMETERS . 7 - 7.6 , ZONAL CURVATURES ARE

10.3 10.6 10.9 11.2 11.55 11.85 12.15 12.5 12.85 13.2 13.55 13.95 14.3 14.7 15.1 15.5 15.9 16.35 16.8

FOR EDGE LIFT 0.07 , OPTIC DIAMETERS 7.2 - 7.8 , ZONAL CURVATURES ARE

10.05 10.35 10.65 10.9 11.2 11.5 11.85 12.15 12.5 12.8 13.15 13.5 13.85 14.25 14.6 15 15.4 15.8 16.2

FOR EDGE LIFT 0.07 , OPTIC DIAMETERS 7.4 - 8 , ZONAL CURVATURES ARE

9.85 10.1 10.35 10.65 10.95 11.25 11.55 11.85 12.15 12.45 12.8 13.1 13.45 13.8 14.15 14.55 14.9 15.3 15.7

FOR EDGE LIFT 0.07 , OPTIC DIAMETERS 7.6 - 8.2 , ZONAL CURVATURES ARE

9.6 9.9 10.15 10.4 10.7 10.95 11.25 11.55 11.85 12.15 12.45 12.75 13.1 13.4 13.75 14.1 14.45 14.85 15.2

FOR EDGE LIFT 0.07 , OPTIC DIAMETERS 7.8 - 8.4 , ZONAL CURVATURES ARE

9.4 9.65 9.9 10.2 10.45 10.7 11 11.25 11.55 11.85 12.15 12.45 12.75 13.05 13.4 13.75 14.05 14.4 14.75

FOR EDGE LIFT 0.07 , OPTIC DIAMETERS 8. - 8.6 , ZONAL CURVATURES ARE

9.25 9.45 9.7 9.95 10.2 10.5 10.75 11 11.3 11.55 11.85 12.15 12.45 12.75 13.05 13.4 13.7 14.05 14.35

FOR EDGE LIFT 0.07 , OPTIC DIAMETERS 8.2 - 8.8 , ZONAL CURVATURES ARE

9.05 9.3 9.55 9.75 10 10.25 10.5 10.8 11.05 11.3 11.6 11.9 12.15 12.45 12.75 13.05 13.35 13.7 14

FOR EDGE LIFT 0.07 , OPTIC DIAMETERS 8.4 - 9 , ZONAL CURVATURES ARE

8.9 9.15 9.35 9.6 9.85 10.05 10.3 10.55 10.85 11.1 11.35 11.65 11.9 12.2 12.45 12.75 13.05 13.35 13.7

FOR EDGE LIFT 0.07 , OPTIC DIAMETERS 8.6 - 9.2 , ZONAL CURVATURES ARE

8.75 8.95 9.2 9.4 9.65 9.9 10.15 10.35 10.6 10.85 11.15 11.4 11.65 11.95 12.2 12.5 12.8 13.05 13.35

FOR EDGE LIFT 0.07 , OPTIC DIAMETERS 8.8 - 9.4 , ZONAL CURVATURES ARE

8.6 8.8 9.05 9.25 9.5 9.7 9.95 10.2 10.45 10.65 10.9 11.15 11.45 11.7 11.95 12.25 12.5 12.8 13.1

FOR EDGE LIFT 0.07 , OPTIC DIAMETERS 9. - 9.6 , ZONAL CURVATURES ARE

8.5 8.7 8.9 9.1 9.35 9.55 9.8 10 10.25 10.5 10.7 10.95 11.2 11.5 11.75 12 12.25 12.55 12.8

FOR EDGE LIFT 0.07 , OPTIC DIAMETERS 9.2 - 9.8 , ZONAL CURVATURES ARE

8.35 8.55 8.75 8.95 9.2 9.4 9.6 9.85 10.05 10.3 10.55 10.8 11 11.25 11.5 11.8 12.05 12.3 12.55

FOR EDGE LIFT 0.07 , OPTIC DIAMETERS 9.4 - 10. , ZONAL CURVATURES ARE

8.25 8.45 8.65 8.85 9.05 9.25 9.45 9.7 9.9 10.15 10.35 10.6 10.85 11.1 11.3 11.55 11.8 12.1 12.35

FOR EDGE LIFT 0.07 , OPTIC DIAMETERS 9.6 - 10.2 , ZONAL CURVATURES ARE

8.15 8.3 8.5 8.7 8.9 9.15 9.35 9.55 9.75 10 10.2 10.45 10.65 10.9 11.15 11.4 11.6 11.85 12.15

FOR EDGE LIFT 0.07 , OPTIC DIAMETERS 9.8 - 10.4 , ZONAL CURVATURES ARE

8.05 8.2 8.4 8.6 8.8 9 9.2 9.4 9.6 9.85 10.05 10.3 10.5 10.75 10.95 11.2 11.45 11.7 11.9

FOR EDGE LIFT 0.07 , OPTIC DIAMETERS 10. - 10.6 , ZONAL CURVATURES ARE

7.95 8.1 8.3 8.5 8.7 8.9 9.1 9.3 9.5 9.7 9.9 10.15 10.35 10.55 10.8 11 11.25 11.5 11.75

FOR EDGE LIFT 0.07 , OPTIC DIAMETERS 10.2 - 10.8 , ZONAL CURVATURES ARE

7.85 8 8.2 8.4 8.6 8.75 8.95 9.15 9.35 9.55 9.75 10 10.2 10.4 10.65 10.85 11.1 11.3 11.55

FOR EDGE LIFT 0.07 , OPTIC DIAMETERS 10.4 - 11. , ZONAL CURVATURES ARE

7.75 7.95 8.1 8.3 8.5 8.65 8.85 9.05 9.25 9.45 9.65 9.85 10.05 10.25 10.5 10.7 10.95 11.15 11.4

```
FOR EDGE LIFT   0.08 ,   OPTIC DIAMETERS   7 - 7.6 ,   ZONAL CURVATURES ARE
 11.2  11.55  11.9  12.3  12.7  13.1  13.5  13.9  14.35  14.8  15.25  15.75  16.25  16.75  17.3  17.85  18.4  19  19.65

FOR EDGE LIFT   0.08 ,   OPTIC DIAMETERS   7.2 - 7.8 ,   ZONAL CURVATURES ARE
 10.85  11.2  11.55  11.9  12.25  12.65  13  13.4  13.85  14.25  14.7  15.15  15.6  16.1  16.55  17.1  17.6  18.15  18.7

FOR EDGE LIFT   0.08 ,   OPTIC DIAMETERS   7.4 - 8 ,   ZONAL CURVATURES ARE
 10.55  10.85  11.2  11.55  11.85  12.25  12.6  12.95  13.35  13.75  14.15  14.6  15  15.45  15.95  16.4  16.9  17.4  17.9

FOR EDGE LIFT   0.08 ,   OPTIC DIAMETERS   7.6 - 8.2 ,   ZONAL CURVATURES ARE
 10.25  10.55  10.9  11.2  11.55  11.85  12.2  12.55  12.95  13.3  13.7  14.1  14.5  14.9  15.35  15.8  16.25  16.75  17.2

FOR EDGE LIFT   0.08 ,   OPTIC DIAMETERS   7.8 - 8.4 ,   ZONAL CURVATURES ARE
 10  10.3  10.6  10.9  11.2  11.55  11.85  12.2  12.55  12.9  13.25  13.65  14.05  14.45  14.85  15.25  15.7  16.15  16.6

FOR EDGE LIFT   0.08 ,   OPTIC DIAMETERS   8. - 8.6 ,   ZONAL CURVATURES ARE
 9.75  10.05  10.35  10.6  10.9  11.25  11.55  11.85  12.2  12.55  12.9  13.25  13.6  14  14.35  14.75  15.15  15.6  16

FOR EDGE LIFT   0.08 ,   OPTIC DIAMETERS   8.2 - 8.8 ,   ZONAL CURVATURES ARE
 9.55  9.8  10.1  10.35  10.65  10.95  11.25  11.55  11.85  12.2  12.55  12.85  13.2  13.6  13.95  14.3  14.7  15.1  15.5

FOR EDGE LIFT   0.08 ,   OPTIC DIAMETERS   8.4 - 9 ,   ZONAL CURVATURES ARE
 9.35  9.6  9.85  10.15  10.4  10.7  11  11.25  11.6  11.9  12.2  12.55  12.85  13.2  13.55  13.9  14.3  14.65  15.05

FOR EDGE LIFT   0.08 ,   OPTIC DIAMETERS   8.6 - 9.2 ,   ZONAL CURVATURES ARE
 9.15  9.4  9.65  9.9  10.2  10.45  10.75  11  11.3  11.6  11.9  12.2  12.55  12.85  13.2  13.55  13.9  14.25  14.6
```

```
FOR EDGE LIFT   0.08 ,   OPTIC DIAMETERS   8.8  -  9.4 ,    ZONAL CURVATURES ARE
 8.95  9.2  9.45  9.7  9.95  10.25  10.5  10.75  11.05  11.35  11.65  11.95  12.25  12.55  12.85  13.2  13.55  13.9  14.25

FOR EDGE LIFT   0.08 ,   OPTIC DIAMETERS   9.  -  9.6 ,    ZONAL CURVATURES ARE
 8.8  9.05  9.25  9.5  9.75  10  10.3  10.55  10.8  11.1  11.4  11.65  11.95  12.25  12.55  12.9  13.2  13.55  13.85

FOR EDGE LIFT   0.08 ,   OPTIC DIAMETERS   9.2  -  9.8 ,    ZONAL CURVATURES ARE
 8.65  8.85  9.1  9.35  9.6  9.85  10.1  10.35  10.6  10.85  11.15  11.4  11.7  12  12.3  12.6  12.9  13.2  13.55

FOR EDGE LIFT   0.08 ,   OPTIC DIAMETERS   9.4  -  10. ,    ZONAL CURVATURES ARE
 8.5  8.7  8.95  9.2  9.4  9.65  9.9  10.15  10.4  10.65  10.9  11.2  11.45  11.75  12.05  12.3  12.6  12.9  13.25

FOR EDGE LIFT   0.08 ,   OPTIC DIAMETERS   9.6  -  10.2 ,    ZONAL CURVATURES ARE
 8.35  8.6  8.8  9  9.25  9.5  9.7  9.95  10.2  10.45  10.7  10.95  11.25  11.5  11.8  12.05  12.35  12.65  12.95

FOR EDGE LIFT   0.08 ,   OPTIC DIAMETERS   9.8  -  10.4 ,    ZONAL CURVATURES ARE
 8.25  8.45  8.65  8.9  9.1  9.3  9.55  9.8  10  10.25  10.5  10.75  11.05  11.3  11.55  11.85  12.1  12.4  12.7

FOR EDGE LIFT   0.08 ,   OPTIC DIAMETERS   10.  -  10.6 ,    ZONAL CURVATURES ARE
 8.1  8.3  8.55  8.75  8.95  9.15  9.4  9.6  9.85  10.1  10.35  10.6  10.85  11.1  11.35  11.6  11.9  12.15  12.45

FOR EDGE LIFT   0.08 ,   OPTIC DIAMETERS   10.2  -  10.8 ,    ZONAL CURVATURES ARE
 8  8.2  8.4  8.6  8.8  9.05  9.25  9.45  9.7  9.95  10.15  10.4  10.65  10.9  11.15  11.4  11.65  11.95  12.2

FOR EDGE LIFT   0.08 ,   OPTIC DIAMETERS   10.4  -  11. ,    ZONAL CURVATURES ARE
 7.9  8.1  8.3  8.5  8.7  8.9  9.1  9.35  9.55  9.75  10  10.25  10.45  10.7  10.95  11.2  11.45  11.7  12
```

FOR EDGE LIFT 0.09 , OPTIC DIAMETERS 7 - 7.6 , ZONAL CURVATURES ARE

12.3 12.7 13.15 13.65 14.15 14.65 15.2 15.75 16.3 16.9 17.55 18.2 18.85 19.6 20.3 21.1 21.95 22.8 23.7

FOR EDGE LIFT 0.09 , OPTIC DIAMETERS 7.2 - 7.8 , ZONAL CURVATURES ARE

11.8 12.25 12.65 13.1 13.55 14 14.5 15 15.55 16.1 16.65 17.25 17.9 18.55 19.2 19.9 20.65 21.4 22.25

FOR EDGE LIFT 0.09 , OPTIC DIAMETERS 7.4 - 8 , ZONAL CURVATURES ARE

11.4 11.8 12.2 12.6 13 13.45 13.9 14.4 14.9 15.4 15.9 16.45 17.05 17.65 18.25 18.9 19.55 20.25 21

FOR EDGE LIFT 0.09 , OPTIC DIAMETERS 7.6 - 8.2 , ZONAL CURVATURES ARE

11 11.4 11.75 12.15 12.55 12.95 13.4 13.85 14.3 14.75 15.25 15.75 16.3 16.85 17.4 18 18.6 19.25 19.9

FOR EDGE LIFT 0.09 , OPTIC DIAMETERS 7.8 - 8.4 , ZONAL CURVATURES ARE

10.7 11.05 11.4 11.75 12.15 12.5 12.9 13.35 13.75 14.2 14.65 15.15 15.65 16.15 16.65 17.2 17.8 18.35 18.95

FOR EDGE LIFT 0.09 , OPTIC DIAMETERS 8. - 8.6 , ZONAL CURVATURES ARE

10.35 10.7 11.05 11.4 11.75 12.1 12.5 12.9 13.3 13.7 14.15 14.6 15.05 15.5 16 16.5 17.05 17.6 18.15

FOR EDGE LIFT 0.09 , OPTIC DIAMETERS 8.2 - 8.8 , ZONAL CURVATURES ARE

10.1 10.4 10.75 11.05 11.4 11.75 12.1 12.5 12.85 13.25 13.65 14.1 14.5 14.95 15.4 15.9 16.4 16.9 17.4

FOR EDGE LIFT 0.09 , OPTIC DIAMETERS 8.4 - 9 , ZONAL CURVATURES ARE

9.85 10.15 10.45 10.75 11.1 11.4 11.75 12.1 12.45 12.85 13.25 13.65 14.05 14.45 14.9 15.35 15.8 16.25 16.75

FOR EDGE LIFT 0.09 , OPTIC DIAMETERS 8.6 - 9.2 , ZONAL CURVATURES ARE

9.6 9.9 10.15 10.45 10.8 11.1 11.45 11.75 12.1 12.45 12.85 13.2 13.6 14 14.4 14.85 15.25 15.7 16.15

```
FOR EDGE LIFT   0.09 ,   OPTIC DIAMETERS   8.8 - 9.4 ,   ZONAL CURVATURES ARE
 9.35  9.65  9.95  10.2  10.5  10.8  11.15  11.45  11.8  12.15  12.5  12.85  13.2  13.6  13.95  14.35  14.8  15.2  15.65

FOR EDGE LIFT   0.09 ,   OPTIC DIAMETERS   9. - 9.6 ,   ZONAL CURVATURES ARE
 9.15  9.45  9.7  10  10.25  10.55  10.85  11.15  11.5  11.8  12.15  12.5  12.85  13.2  13.55  13.95  14.35  14.75  15.15

FOR EDGE LIFT   0.09 ,   OPTIC DIAMETERS   9.2 - 9.8 ,   ZONAL CURVATURES ARE
 8.95  9.25  9.5  9.75  10.05  10.3  10.6  10.9  11.2  11.5  11.85  12.15  12.5  12.85  13.2  13.55  13.95  14.3  14.7

FOR EDGE LIFT   0.09 ,   OPTIC DIAMETERS   9.4 - 10. ,   ZONAL CURVATURES ARE
 8.8  9.05  9.3  9.55  9.8  10.1  10.35  10.65  10.95  11.25  11.55  11.85  12.2  12.5  12.85  13.2  13.55  13.9  14.3

FOR EDGE LIFT   0.09 ,   OPTIC DIAMETERS   9.6 - 10.2 ,   ZONAL CURVATURES ARE
 8.65  8.85  9.1  9.35  9.6  9.9  10.15  10.4  10.7  11  11.3  11.6  11.9  12.2  12.55  12.85  13.2  13.55  13.9

FOR EDGE LIFT   0.09 ,   OPTIC DIAMETERS   9.8 - 10.4 ,   ZONAL CURVATURES ARE
 8.45  8.7  8.95  9.2  9.45  9.7  9.95  10.2  10.5  10.75  11.05  11.35  11.65  11.95  12.25  12.55  12.9  13.25  13.55

FOR EDGE LIFT   0.09 ,   OPTIC DIAMETERS   10. - 10.6 ,   ZONAL CURVATURES ARE
 8.35  8.55  8.8  9  9.25  9.5  9.75  10  10.25  10.55  10.8  11.1  11.4  11.7  12  12.3  12.6  12.9  13.25

FOR EDGE LIFT   0.09 ,   OPTIC DIAMETERS   10.2 - 10.8 ,   ZONAL CURVATURES ARE
 8.2  8.4  8.65  8.85  9.1  9.35  9.55  9.8  10.1  10.35  10.6  10.85  11.15  11.45  11.7  12  12.3  12.65  12.95

FOR EDGE LIFT   0.09 ,   OPTIC DIAMETERS   10.4 - 11. ,   ZONAL CURVATURES ARE
 8.05  8.3  8.5  8.7  8.95  9.15  9.4  9.65  9.9  10.15  10.4  10.65  10.95  11.2  11.5  11.75  12.05  12.35  12.65
```

```
FOR EDGE LIFT   0.1 ,   OPTIC DIAMETERS   7  -  7.6 ,    ZONAL CURVATURES ARE
 13.65  14.2  14.75  15.4  16.05  16.7  17.4  18.15  18.95  19.8  20.65  21.6  22.55  23.6  24.75  25.9  27.2  28.55  30

FOR EDGE LIFT   0.1 ,   OPTIC DIAMETERS   7.2  -  7.8 ,    ZONAL CURVATURES ARE
 13  13.5  14.05  14.6  15.2  15.8  16.45  17.1  17.85  18.55  19.35  20.2  21.05  21.95  22.95  23.95  25.05  26.25  27.45

FOR EDGE LIFT   0.1 ,   OPTIC DIAMETERS   7.4  -  8 ,    ZONAL CURVATURES ARE
 12.45  12.9  13.4  13.95  14.45  15.05  15.6  16.25  16.85  17.55  18.25  19  19.75  20.6  21.45  22.35  23.3  24.35  25.4

FOR EDGE LIFT   0.1 ,   OPTIC DIAMETERS   7.6  -  8.2 ,    ZONAL CURVATURES ARE
 11.95  12.4  12.85  13.35  13.85  14.35  14.9  15.45  16.05  16.65  17.3  17.95  18.65  19.4  20.2  21  21.85  22.75  23.7

FOR EDGE LIFT   0.1 ,   OPTIC DIAMETERS   7.8  -  8.4 ,    ZONAL CURVATURES ARE
 11.5  11.9  12.35  12.8  13.25  13.75  14.25  14.75  15.3  15.85  16.45  17.05  17.7  18.4  19.1  19.8  20.6  21.4  22.25

FOR EDGE LIFT   0.1 ,   OPTIC DIAMETERS   8.  -  8.6 ,    ZONAL CURVATURES ARE
 11.1  11.5  11.9  12.3  12.75  13.2  13.65  14.15  14.65  15.2  15.7  16.3  16.9  17.5  18.15  18.8  19.5  20.25  21

FOR EDGE LIFT   0.1 ,   OPTIC DIAMETERS   8.2  -  8.8 ,    ZONAL CURVATURES ARE
 10.75  11.1  11.5  11.9  12.3  12.7  13.15  13.6  14.1  14.55  15.05  15.6  16.15  16.7  17.3  17.9  18.55  19.25  19.9

FOR EDGE LIFT   0.1 ,   OPTIC DIAMETERS   8.4  -  9 ,    ZONAL CURVATURES ARE
 10.4  10.75  11.1  11.5  11.9  12.3  12.7  13.1  13.55  14  14.5  15  15.5  16  16.55  17.15  17.7  18.35  19

FOR EDGE LIFT   0.1 ,   OPTIC DIAMETERS   8.6  -  9.2 ,    ZONAL CURVATURES ARE
 10.1  10.45  10.8  11.15  11.5  11.9  12.25  12.65  13.1  13.5  13.95  14.4  14.9  15.4  15.9  16.45  17  17.55  18.15
```

```
FOR EDGE LIFT   0.1 ,   OPTIC DIAMETERS   8.8  -  9.4 ,    ZONAL CURVATURES ARE
 9.85  10.15  10.45  10.8  11.15  11.5  11.9  12.25  12.65  13.05  13.5  13.9  14.35  14.85  15.3  15.8  16.3  16.85  17.4

FOR EDGE LIFT   0.1 ,   OPTIC DIAMETERS   9.  -  9.6 ,    ZONAL CURVATURES ARE
 9.55  9.85  10.2  10.5  10.85  11.2  11.55  11.9  12.25  12.65  13.05  13.45  13.9  14.3  14.75  15.25  15.7  16.2  16.75

FOR EDGE LIFT   0.1 ,   OPTIC DIAMETERS   9.2  -  9.8 ,    ZONAL CURVATURES ARE
 9.35  9.65  9.95  10.25  10.55  10.9  11.2  11.55  11.9  12.3  12.65  13.05  13.45  13.85  14.3  14.75  15.2  15.65  16.15

FOR EDGE LIFT   0.1 ,   OPTIC DIAMETERS   9.4  -  10. ,    ZONAL CURVATURES ARE
 9.1  9.4  9.7  10  10.3  10.6  10.9  11.25  11.6  11.95  12.3  12.65  13.05  13.45  13.85  14.25  14.7  15.15  15.6

FOR EDGE LIFT   0.1 ,   OPTIC DIAMETERS   9.6  -  10.2 ,    ZONAL CURVATURES ARE
 8.9  9.2  9.45  9.75  10.05  10.35  10.65  10.95  11.3  11.6  11.95  12.3  12.7  13.05  13.45  13.85  14.25  14.65  15.1

FOR EDGE LIFT   0.1 ,   OPTIC DIAMETERS   9.8  -  10.4 ,    ZONAL CURVATURES ARE
 8.75  9  9.25  9.55  9.8  10.1  10.4  10.7  11  11.3  11.65  12  12.35  12.7  13.05  13.45  13.85  14.25  14.65

FOR EDGE LIFT   0.1 ,   OPTIC DIAMETERS   10.  -  10.6 ,    ZONAL CURVATURES ARE
 8.55  8.8  9.05  9.3  9.6  9.85  10.15  10.45  10.75  11.05  11.35  11.7  12  12.35  12.7  13.1  13.45  13.85  14.2

FOR EDGE LIFT   0.1 ,   OPTIC DIAMETERS   10.2  -  10.8 ,    ZONAL CURVATURES ARE
 8.4  8.65  8.9  9.15  9.4  9.65  9.95  10.2  10.5  10.8  11.1  11.4  11.75  12.05  12.4  12.75  13.1  13.45  13.85

FOR EDGE LIFT   0.1 ,   OPTIC DIAMETERS   10.4  -  11. ,    ZONAL CURVATURES ARE
 8.25  8.5  8.7  8.95  9.2  9.45  9.75  10  10.3  10.55  10.85  11.15  11.45  11.75  12.1  12.45  12.75  13.1  13.45
```

FOR EDGE LIFT 0.11 , OPTIC DIAMETERS 7 - 7.6 , ZONAL CURVATURES ARE

15.35 16.1 16.85 17.7 18.55 19.5 20.5 21.55 22.7 23.9 25.25 26.65 28.2 29.85 31.7 33.7 35.9 38.35 41.05

FOR EDGE LIFT 0.11 , OPTIC DIAMETERS 7.2 - 7.8 , ZONAL CURVATURES ARE

14.5 15.15 15.85 16.55 17.35 18.15 19.05 20 20.95 22 23.15 24.35 25.65 27.05 28.6 30.2 32 33.95 36.1

FOR EDGE LIFT 0.11 , OPTIC DIAMETERS 7.4 - 8 , ZONAL CURVATURES ARE

13.75 14.35 14.95 15.6 16.3 17.05 17.85 18.65 19.55 20.45 21.45 22.5 23.6 24.8 26.1 27.5 28.95 30.6 32.3

FOR EDGE LIFT 0.11 , OPTIC DIAMETERS 7.6 - 8.2 , ZONAL CURVATURES ARE

13.05 13.6 14.2 14.8 15.45 16.1 16.8 17.55 18.3 19.15 20 20.95 21.9 22.95 24.1 25.25 26.55 27.9 29.35

FOR EDGE LIFT 0.11 , OPTIC DIAMETERS 7.8 - 8.4 , ZONAL CURVATURES ARE

12.5 13 13.5 14.1 14.65 15.25 15.9 16.6 17.3 18 18.8 19.65 20.5 21.4 22.4 23.45 24.55 25.7 27

FOR EDGE LIFT 0.11 , OPTIC DIAMETERS 8. - 8.6 , ZONAL CURVATURES ARE

11.95 12.45 12.95 13.45 14 14.55 15.1 15.75 16.4 17.05 17.75 18.5 19.3 20.1 21 21.9 22.9 23.9 25

FOR EDGE LIFT 0.11 , OPTIC DIAMETERS 8.2 - 8.8 , ZONAL CURVATURES ARE

11.5 11.95 12.4 12.85 13.35 13.9 14.45 15 15.6 16.2 16.85 17.55 18.25 19 19.75 20.6 21.45 22.4 23.35

FOR EDGE LIFT 0.11 , OPTIC DIAMETERS 8.4 - 9 , ZONAL CURVATURES ARE

11.1 11.5 11.9 12.35 12.85 13.3 13.8 14.35 14.9 15.45 16.05 16.7 17.35 18 18.7 19.45 20.25 21.1 21.95

FOR EDGE LIFT 0.11 , OPTIC DIAMETERS 8.6 - 9.2 , ZONAL CURVATURES ARE

10.7 11.1 11.5 11.9 12.35 12.8 13.25 13.75 14.25 14.8 15.35 15.9 16.5 17.15 17.8 18.5 19.2 19.95 20.75

```
FOR EDGE LIFT   0.11 ,   OPTIC DIAMETERS   8.8  -  9.4 ,    ZONAL CURVATURES ARE
 10.35  10.7  11.1  11.5  11.9  12.35  12.8  13.25  13.7  14.2  14.7  15.25  15.8  16.4  17  17.6  18.3  18.95  19.7

FOR EDGE LIFT   0.11 ,   OPTIC DIAMETERS   9.  -  9.6 ,    ZONAL CURVATURES ARE
 10.05  10.4  10.75  11.15  11.5  11.9  12.35  12.75  13.2  13.65  14.15  14.65  15.15  15.7  16.25  16.85  17.45  18.1  18.75

FOR EDGE LIFT   0.11 ,   OPTIC DIAMETERS   9.2  -  9.8 ,    ZONAL CURVATURES ARE
 9.75  10.1  10.45  10.8  11.15  11.55  11.9  12.35  12.75  13.2  13.65  14.1  14.6  15.1  15.6  16.15  16.75  17.3  17.95

FOR EDGE LIFT   0.11 ,   OPTIC DIAMETERS   9.4  -  10. ,    ZONAL CURVATURES ARE
 9.5  9.8  10.15  10.45  10.8  11.2  11.55  11.95  12.35  12.75  13.15  13.6  14.05  14.55  15.05  15.55  16.1  16.6  17.2

FOR EDGE LIFT   0.11 ,   OPTIC DIAMETERS   9.6  -  10.2 ,    ZONAL CURVATURES ARE
 9.25  9.55  9.85  10.2  10.5  10.85  11.2  11.6  11.95  12.35  12.75  13.15  13.6  14.05  14.5  15  15.5  16  16.55

FOR EDGE LIFT   0.11 ,   OPTIC DIAMETERS   9.8  -  10.4 ,    ZONAL CURVATURES ARE
 9  9.3  9.6  9.9  10.25  10.55  10.9  11.25  11.6  12  12.35  12.75  13.15  13.6  14.05  14.5  14.95  15.45  15.95

FOR EDGE LIFT   0.11 ,   OPTIC DIAMETERS   10.  -  10.6 ,    ZONAL CURVATURES ARE
 8.8  9.1  9.35  9.65  9.95  10.3  10.6  10.95  11.3  11.65  12  12.4  12.75  13.15  13.6  14  14.45  14.9  15.4

FOR EDGE LIFT   0.11 ,   OPTIC DIAMETERS   10.2  -  10.8 ,    ZONAL CURVATURES ARE
 8.6  8.9  9.15  9.45  9.75  10.05  10.35  10.65  11  11.35  11.65  12.05  12.4  12.8  13.2  13.6  14  14.45  14.9

FOR EDGE LIFT   0.11 ,   OPTIC DIAMETERS   10.4  -  11. ,    ZONAL CURVATURES ARE
 8.45  8.7  8.95  9.25  9.5  9.8  10.1  10.4  10.7  11.05  11.35  11.7  12.05  12.45  12.8  13.2  13.6  14  14.45
```

```
FOR EDGE LIFT   0.12 ,   OPTIC DIAMETERS   7 - 7.6 ,    ZONAL CURVATURES ARE
 17.65  18.65  19.7  20.9  22.15  23.5  25  26.6  28.4  30.35  32.55  35  37.7  40.8  44.35  48.4  53.15  58.7  65.35

FOR EDGE LIFT   0.12 ,   OPTIC DIAMETERS   7.2 - 7.8 ,    ZONAL CURVATURES ARE
 16.4  17.3  18.2  19.2  20.3  21.45  22.7  24.05  25.55  27.15  28.9  30.85  33  35.4  38.05  41.05  44.45  48.35  52.85

FOR EDGE LIFT   0.12 ,   OPTIC DIAMETERS   7.4 - 8 ,    ZONAL CURVATURES ARE
 15.35  16.15  16.95  17.85  18.8  19.8  20.85  22  23.3  24.65  26.1  27.7  29.45  31.35  33.45  35.8  38.4  41.3  44.6

FOR EDGE LIFT   0.12 ,   OPTIC DIAMETERS   7.6 - 8.2 ,    ZONAL CURVATURES ARE
 14.45  15.15  15.9  16.7  17.5  18.4  19.35  20.35  21.45  22.6  23.85  25.2  26.65  28.25  29.95  31.85  33.95  36.25  38.75

FOR EDGE LIFT   0.12 ,   OPTIC DIAMETERS   7.8 - 8.4 ,    ZONAL CURVATURES ARE
 13.7  14.3  15  15.7  16.45  17.25  18.05  18.95  19.9  20.9  22  23.15  24.4  25.75  27.2  28.8  30.5  32.35  34.4

FOR EDGE LIFT   0.12 ,   OPTIC DIAMETERS   8. - 8.6 ,    ZONAL CURVATURES ARE
 13  13.6  14.2  14.85  15.5  16.25  17  17.8  18.6  19.5  20.5  21.5  22.6  23.75  25  26.35  27.8  29.35  31.05

FOR EDGE LIFT   0.12 ,   OPTIC DIAMETERS   8.2 - 8.8 ,    ZONAL CURVATURES ARE
 12.4  12.95  13.5  14.1  14.7  15.35  16.05  16.75  17.5  18.35  19.2  20.1  21.05  22.05  23.15  24.3  25.55  26.9  28.35

FOR EDGE LIFT   0.12 ,   OPTIC DIAMETERS   8.4 - 9 ,    ZONAL CURVATURES ARE
 11.9  12.35  12.9  13.45  14  14.6  15.2  15.85  16.55  17.3  18.05  18.85  19.75  20.65  21.6  22.65  23.75  24.9  26.15

FOR EDGE LIFT   0.12 ,   OPTIC DIAMETERS   8.6 - 9.2 ,    ZONAL CURVATURES ARE
 11.4  11.85  12.35  12.85  13.35  13.9  14.5  15.1  15.75  16.4  17.1  17.85  18.6  19.45  20.3  21.2  22.15  23.2  24.3
```

FOR EDGE LIFT 0.12 , OPTIC DIAMETERS 8.8 - 9.4 , ZONAL CURVATURES ARE

10.95 11.4 11.85 12.3 12.8 13.3 13.85 14.4 15 15.6 16.25 16.9 17.65 18.35 19.15 20 20.85 21.75 22.75

FOR EDGE LIFT 0.12 , OPTIC DIAMETERS 9. - 9.6 , ZONAL CURVATURES ARE

10.6 11 11.4 11.85 12.3 12.8 13.3 13.8 14.35 14.9 15.5 16.1 16.75 17.45 18.15 18.9 19.7 20.55 21.4

FOR EDGE LIFT 0.12 , OPTIC DIAMETERS 9.2 - 9.8 , ZONAL CURVATURES ARE

10.25 10.6 11 11.4 11.85 12.3 12.75 13.25 13.75 14.3 14.85 15.4 16 16.65 17.3 17.95 18.7 19.45 20.25

FOR EDGE LIFT 0.12 , OPTIC DIAMETERS 9.4 - 10. , ZONAL CURVATURES ARE

9.9 10.25 10.65 11.05 11.45 11.35 12.3 12.75 13.2 13.7 14.25 14.75 15.3 15.9 16.5 17.15 17.8 18.5 19.25

FOR EDGE LIFT 0.12 , OPTIC DIAMETERS 9.6 - 10.2 , ZONAL CURVATURES ARE

9.6 9.95 10.3 10.7 11.05 11.45 11.85 12.3 12.75 13.2 13.7 14.2 14.7 15.25 15.8 16.4 17 17.65 18.35

FOR EDGE LIFT 0.12 , OPTIC DIAMETERS 9.8 - 10.4 , ZONAL CURVATURES ARE

9.35 9.65 10 10.35 10.7 11.1 11.5 11.9 12.3 12.75 13.2 13.65 14.15 14.65 15.2 15.75 16.3 16.9 17.5

FOR EDGE LIFT 0.12 , OPTIC DIAMETERS 10. - 10.6 , ZONAL CURVATURES ARE

9.1 9.4 9.7 10.05 10.4 10.75 11.15 11.5 11.9 12.3 12.75 13.2 13.65 14.15 14.6 15.15 15.65 16.25 16.8

FOR EDGE LIFT 0.12 , OPTIC DIAMETERS 10.2 - 10.8 , ZONAL CURVATURES ARE

8.85 9.15 9.45 9.8 10.1 10.45 10.8 11.15 11.55 11.95 12.35 12.75 13.2 13.65 14.1 14.6 15.1 15.6 16.15

FOR EDGE LIFT 0.12 , OPTIC DIAMETERS 10.4 - 11. , ZONAL CURVATURES ARE

8.65 8.95 9.25 9.55 9.85 10.15 10.5 10.85 11.2 11.6 11.95 12.35 12.75 13.2 13.65 14.1 14.55 15.05 15.55

```
FOR EDGE LIFT   0.13 ,   OPTIC DIAMETERS   7 - 7.6 ,   ZONAL CURVATURES ARE
 20.85  22.25  23.85  25.55  27.5  29.65  32.1  34.9  38.05  41.75  46.05  51.15  57.25  64.8  74.2  86.45 NE  NE  NE

FOR EDGE LIFT   0.13 ,   OPTIC DIAMETERS   7.2 - 7.8 ,   ZONAL CURVATURES ARE
 19  20.2  21.5  22.95  24.55  26.25  28.2  30.35  32.8  35.55  38.65  42.25  46.4  51.35  57.2  64.35  73.15  84.45 NE

FOR EDGE LIFT   0.13 ,   OPTIC DIAMETERS   7.4 - 8 ,   ZONAL CURVATURES ARE
 17.5  18.55  19.65  20.85  22.2  23.65  25.25  26.95  28.9  31.05  33.45  36.15  39.25  42.75  46.85  51.6  57.25  64  72.3

FOR EDGE LIFT   0.13 ,   OPTIC DIAMETERS   7.6 - 8.2 ,   ZONAL CURVATURES ARE
 16.25  17.15  18.15  19.2  20.3  21.55  22.9  24.35  25.95  27.7  29.6  31.75  34.15  36.8  39.85  43.3  47.25  51.9  57.3

FOR EDGE LIFT   0.13 ,   OPTIC DIAMETERS   7.8 - 8.4 ,   ZONAL CURVATURES ARE
 15.2  16  16.85  17.8  18.8  19.85  21  22.25  23.55  25.05  26.65  28.4  30.3  32.45  34.8  37.45  40.45  43.85  47.7

FOR EDGE LIFT   0.13 ,   OPTIC DIAMETERS   8. - 8.6 ,   ZONAL CURVATURES ARE
 14.3  15  15.8  16.6  17.5  18.4  19.4  20.5  21.65  22.9  24.25  25.75  27.35  29.1  31  33.15  35.5  38.1  41.05

FOR EDGE LIFT   0.13 ,   OPTIC DIAMETERS   8.2 - 8.8 ,   ZONAL CURVATURES ARE
 13.5  14.15  14.85  15.6  16.4  17.2  18.1  19.05  20.05  21.15  22.3  23.6  24.95  26.4  28.05  29.8  31.7  33.8  36.15

FOR EDGE LIFT   0.13 ,   OPTIC DIAMETERS   8.4 - 9 ,   ZONAL CURVATURES ARE
 12.85  13.45  14.05  14.75  15.45  16.2  17  17.85  18.75  19.7  20.7  21.8  23  24.25  25.65  27.1  28.75  30.5  32.4

FOR EDGE LIFT   0.13 ,   OPTIC DIAMETERS   8.6 - 9.2 ,   ZONAL CURVATURES ARE
 12.25  12.8  13.35  13.95  14.6  15.3  16  16.8  17.6  18.45  19.35  20.35  21.35  22.45  23.65  24.95  26.3  27.8  29.45
```

```
FOR EDGE LIFT   0.13 ,   OPTIC DIAMETERS   8.8  -  9.4 ,    ZONAL CURVATURES ARE
 11.7  12.2  12.75  13.3  13.9  14.5  15.15  15.85  16.6  17.35  18.2  19.05  20  20.95  22  23.15  24.35  25.65  27

FOR EDGE LIFT   0.13 ,   OPTIC DIAMETERS   9.  -  9.6 ,    ZONAL CURVATURES ARE
 11.2  11.7  12.2  12.7  13.25  13.8  14.4  15.05  15.75  16.45  17.15  17.95  18.8  19.65  20.6  21.6  22.65  23.8  25

FOR EDGE LIFT   0.13 ,   OPTIC DIAMETERS   9.2  -  9.8 ,    ZONAL CURVATURES ARE
 10.75  11.2  11.7  12.15  12.65  13.2  13.75  14.35  14.95  15.6  16.3  17  17.75  18.55  19.4  20.3  21.25  22.25  23.3

FOR EDGE LIFT   0.13 ,   OPTIC DIAMETERS   9.4  -  10. ,    ZONAL CURVATURES ARE
 10.4  10.8  11.25  11.7  12.15  12.65  13.15  13.7  14.3  14.9  15.5  16.15  16.85  17.6  18.35  19.15  20  20.9  21.9

FOR EDGE LIFT   0.13 ,   OPTIC DIAMETERS   9.6  -  10.2 ,    ZONAL CURVATURES ARE
 10.05  10.4  10.85  11.25  11.7  12.15  12.65  13.15  13.7  14.25  14.8  15.4  16.05  16.7  17.4  18.15  18.95  19.75  20.65

FOR EDGE LIFT   0.13 ,   OPTIC DIAMETERS   9.8  -  10.4 ,    ZONAL CURVATURES ARE
 9.7  10.05  10.45  10.85  11.3  11.7  12.15  12.65  13.15  13.65  14.2  14.75  15.35  15.95  16.6  17.3  18  18.75  19.55

FOR EDGE LIFT   0.13 ,   OPTIC DIAMETERS   10.  -  10.6 ,    ZONAL CURVATURES ARE
 9.4  9.75  10.1  10.5  10.9  11.3  11.75  12.15  12.65  13.1  13.6  14.15  14.7  15.25  15.85  16.5  17.15  17.85  18.55

FOR EDGE LIFT   0.13 ,   OPTIC DIAMETERS   10.2  -  10.8 ,    ZONAL CURVATURES ARE
 9.15  9.45  9.8  10.15  10.55  10.95  11.35  11.75  12.2  12.65  13.1  13.6  14.1  14.65  15.2  15.8  16.4  17.05  17.7

FOR EDGE LIFT   0.13 ,   OPTIC DIAMETERS   10.4  -  11. ,    ZONAL CURVATURES ARE
 8.9  9.2  9.55  9.85  10.25  10.6  10.95  11.35  11.8  12.2  12.65  13.1  13.6  14.1  14.6  15.15  15.75  16.35  16.95
```

```
FOR EDGE LIFT   0.14 ,   OPTIC DIAMETERS   7  -  7.6 ,    ZONAL CURVATURES ARE
 25.5  27.7  30.2  33.1  36.5  40.45  45.2  50.95  58.05 NE  NE  NE  NE  NE  NE  NE  NE  NE  NE

FOR EDGE LIFT   0.14 ,   OPTIC DIAMETERS   7.2  -  7.8 ,    ZONAL CURVATURES ARE
 22.65  24.4  26.35  28.6  31.1  34.05  37.4  41.3  46  51.65  58.6 NE  NE  NE  NE  NE  NE  NE  NE

FOR EDGE LIFT   0.14 ,   OPTIC DIAMETERS   7.4  -  8 ,    ZONAL CURVATURES ARE
 20.4  21.85  23.45  25.25  27.25  29.5  32.05  34.95  38.3  42.2  46.8  52.35  59.15 NE  NE  NE  NE  NE  NE

FOR EDGE LIFT   0.14 ,   OPTIC DIAMETERS   7.6  -  8.2 ,    ZONAL CURVATURES ARE
 18.6  19.85  21.2  22.65  24.3  26.1  28.1  30.4  32.95  35.85  39.2  43.1  47.65  53.1  59.7 NE  NE  NE  NE

FOR EDGE LIFT   0.14 ,   OPTIC DIAMETERS   7.8  -  8.4 ,    ZONAL CURVATURES ARE
 17.15  18.2  19.35  20.6  21.95  23.45  25.1  26.95  29  31.25  33.85  36.75  40.1  43.95  48.5  53.85  60.3 NE  NE

FOR EDGE LIFT   0.14 ,   OPTIC DIAMETERS   8.  -  8.6 ,    ZONAL CURVATURES ARE
 15.95  16.85  17.85  18.95  20.1  21.4  22.75  24.3  25.95  27.8  29.85  32.15  34.75  37.65  41  44.85  49.35  54.6  60.95

FOR EDGE LIFT   0.14 ,   OPTIC DIAMETERS   8.2  -  8.8 ,    ZONAL CURVATURES ARE
 14.9  15.7  16.6  17.55  18.55  19.65  20.85  22.15  23.55  25.1  26.8  28.65  30.75  33.05  35.65  38.6  41.9  45.75  50.15

FOR EDGE LIFT   0.14 ,   OPTIC DIAMETERS   8.4  -  9 ,    ZONAL CURVATURES ARE
 14  14.75  15.5  16.35  17.25  18.25  19.3  20.4  21.6  22.95  24.35  25.95  27.65  29.55  31.65  33.95  36.55  39.5  42.8

FOR EDGE LIFT   0.14 ,   OPTIC DIAMETERS   8.6  -  9.2 ,    ZONAL CURVATURES ARE
 13.2  13.9  14.6  15.35  16.15  17.05  17.95  18.95  20  21.15  22.35  23.7  25.15  26.75  28.5  30.4  32.5  34.85  37.45
```

```
FOR EDGE LIFT   0.14 ,   OPTIC DIAMETERS   8.8  -  9.4 ,    ZONAL CURVATURES ARE
 12.55  13.15  13.8  14.5  15.2  16  16.8  17.7  18.65  19.65  20.7  21.9  23.15  24.5  25.95  27.6  29.35  31.25  33.4

FOR EDGE LIFT   0.14 ,   OPTIC DIAMETERS   9.  -  9.6 ,    ZONAL CURVATURES ARE
 11.95  12.5  13.1  13.7  14.4  15.1  15.85  16.6  17.45  18.35  19.3  20.35  21.45  22.65  23.9  25.3  26.8  28.4  30.2

FOR EDGE LIFT   0.14 ,   OPTIC DIAMETERS   9.2  -  9.8 ,    ZONAL CURVATURES ARE
 11.4  11.95  12.5  13.05  13.65  14.3  15  15.7  16.45  17.25  18.15  19.05  20  21.05  22.2  23.4  24.7  26.1  27.6

FOR EDGE LIFT   0.14 ,   OPTIC DIAMETERS   9.4  -  10. ,    ZONAL CURVATURES ARE
 10.95  11.4  11.9  12.45  13  13.6  14.25  14.9  15.6  16.3  17.1  17.9  18.8  19.75  20.7  21.8  22.9  24.15  25.45

FOR EDGE LIFT   0.14 ,   OPTIC DIAMETERS   9.6  -  10.2 ,    ZONAL CURVATURES ARE
 10.5  10.95  11.4  11.9  12.45  13  13.55  14.15  14.8  15.45  16.2  16.95  17.75  18.55  19.45  20.4  21.45  22.5  23.65

FOR EDGE LIFT   0.14 ,   OPTIC DIAMETERS   9.8  -  10.4 ,    ZONAL CURVATURES ARE
 10.1  10.55  11  11.45  11.9  12.45  12.95  13.5  14.1  14.75  15.4  16.05  16.8  17.55  18.35  19.25  20.15  21.1  22.15

FOR EDGE LIFT   0.14 ,   OPTIC DIAMETERS   10.  -  10.6 ,    ZONAL CURVATURES ARE
 9.75  10.15  10.55  11  11.45  11.95  12.45  12.95  13.5  14.05  14.65  15.3  15.95  16.65  17.4  18.2  19  19.9  20.8

FOR EDGE LIFT   0.14 ,   OPTIC DIAMETERS   10.2  -  10.8 ,    ZONAL CURVATURES ARE
 9.45  9.8  10.2  10.6  11.05  11.5  11.95  12.45  12.95  13.45  14.05  14.6  15.25  15.9  16.55  17.3  18.05  18.85  19.65

FOR EDGE LIFT   0.14 ,   OPTIC DIAMETERS   10.4  -  11. ,    ZONAL CURVATURES ARE
 9.15  9.5  9.85  10.25  10.65  11.05  11.5  11.95  12.45  12.95  13.45  14  14.55  15.15  15.8  16.45  17.15  17.9  18.65
```

```
FOR EDGE LIFT   0.15 ,   OPTIC DIAMETERS   7  -  7.6 ,   ZONAL CURVATURES ARE
 33  36.85  41.5  47.2  54.4  63.85 NE  NE  NE  NE  NE  NE  NE  NE  NE  NE  NE  NE  NE

FOR EDGE LIFT   0.15 ,   OPTIC DIAMETERS   7.2  -  7.8 ,   ZONAL CURVATURES ARE
 28.1  30.9  34.2  38.1  42.75  48.5  55.7 NE  NE  NE  NE  NE  NE  NE  NE  NE  NE  NE  NE

FOR EDGE LIFT   0.15 ,   OPTIC DIAMETERS   7.4  -  8 ,   ZONAL CURVATURES ARE
 24.55  26.7  29.2  32.05  35.4  39.3  44.05  49.8  57 NE  NE  NE  NE  NE  NE  NE  NE  NE  NE

FOR EDGE LIFT   0.15 ,   OPTIC DIAMETERS   7.6  -  8.2 ,   ZONAL CURVATURES ARE
 21.85  23.6  25.55  27.75  30.3  33.2  36.6  40.55  45.35  51.1  58.25 NE  NE  NE  NE  NE  NE  NE  NE

FOR EDGE LIFT   0.15 ,   OPTIC DIAMETERS   7.8  -  8.4 ,   ZONAL CURVATURES ARE
 19.75  21.2  22.8  24.55  26.6  28.85  31.4  34.35  37.8  41.8  46.6  52.4  59.55 NE  NE  NE  NE  NE  NE

FOR EDGE LIFT   0.15 ,   OPTIC DIAMETERS   8.  -  8.6 ,   ZONAL CURVATURES ARE
 18.05  19.25  20.6  22.1  23.75  25.55  27.6  29.9  32.55  35.55  39  43.1  47.9  53.7  60.8 NE  NE  NE  NE

FOR EDGE LIFT   0.15 ,   OPTIC DIAMETERS   8.2  -  8.8 ,   ZONAL CURVATURES ARE
 16.6  17.7  18.85  20.1  21.5  23  24.7  26.55  28.65  31  33.65  36.7  40.25  44.35  49.2  55  62.1 NE  NE

FOR EDGE LIFT   0.15 ,   OPTIC DIAMETERS   8.4  -  9 ,   ZONAL CURVATURES ARE
 15.45  16.35  17.4  18.45  19.65  20.95  22.35  23.9  25.65  27.55  29.7  32.1  34.8  37.9  41.45  45.6  50.45  56.3  63.4

FOR EDGE LIFT   0.15 ,   OPTIC DIAMETERS   8.6  -  9.2 ,   ZONAL CURVATURES ARE
 14.45  15.25  16.15  17.1  18.15  19.25  20.5  21.8  23.25  24.85  26.6  28.55  30.75  33.2  35.95  39.05  42.65  46.85  51.75
```

```
FOR EDGE LIFT   0.15 ,   OPTIC DIAMETERS   8.8  -  9.4 ,    ZONAL CURVATURES ARE
 13.55  14.3  15.1  15.95  16.85  17.85  18.9  20.05  21.3  22.7  24.15  25.8  27.6  29.6  31.8  34.3  37.05  40.25  43.9

FOR EDGE LIFT   0.15 ,   OPTIC DIAMETERS   9.  -  9.6 ,    ZONAL CURVATURES ARE
 12.8  13.5  14.2  14.95  15.8  16.65  17.6  18.6  19.7  20.9  22.15  23.55  25.05  26.75  28.55  30.6  32.85  35.4  38.2

FOR EDGE LIFT   0.15 ,   OPTIC DIAMETERS   9.2  -  9.8 ,    ZONAL CURVATURES ARE
 12.15  12.75  13.4  14.1  14.85  15.65  16.5  17.4  18.35  19.4  20.5  21.7  23  24.45  26  27.7  29.55  31.65  33.95

FOR EDGE LIFT   0.15 ,   OPTIC DIAMETERS   9.4  -  10. ,    ZONAL CURVATURES ARE
 11.55  12.15  12.75  13.35  14.05  14.75  15.5  16.3  17.2  18.1  19.1  20.15  21.3  22.55  23.9  25.35  26.9  28.65  30.55

FOR EDGE LIFT   0.15 ,   OPTIC DIAMETERS   9.6  -  10.2 ,    ZONAL CURVATURES ARE
 11.05  11.55  12.1  12.7  13.3  13.95  14.65  15.4  16.15  17  17.9  18.85  19.85  20.95  22.1  23.4  24.75  26.25  27.85

FOR EDGE LIFT   0.15 ,   OPTIC DIAMETERS   9.8  -  10.4 ,    ZONAL CURVATURES ARE
 10.6  11.05  11.6  12.1  12.7  13.3  13.9  14.6  15.3  16.05  16.85  17.7  18.6  19.6  20.6  21.75  22.95  24.25  25.65

FOR EDGE LIFT   0.15 ,   OPTIC DIAMETERS   10.  -  10.6 ,    ZONAL CURVATURES ARE
 10.15  10.6  11.1  11.6  12.1  12.65  13.25  13.85  14.5  15.2  15.95  16.7  17.55  18.4  19.35  20.35  21.4  22.55  23.75

FOR EDGE LIFT   0.15 ,   OPTIC DIAMETERS   10.2  -  10.8 ,    ZONAL CURVATURES ARE
 9.8  10.2  10.65  11.1  11.6  12.1  12.65  13.2  13.8  14.45  15.1  15.85  16.6  17.35  18.2  19.1  20.05  21.1  22.2

FOR EDGE LIFT   0.15 ,   OPTIC DIAMETERS   10.4  -  11. ,    ZONAL CURVATURES ARE
 9.45  9.85  10.25  10.7  11.15  11.6  12.1  12.65  13.2  13.8  14.4  15.05  15.75  16.45  17.25  18.05  18.9  19.85  20.8
```

TABLE VI Back Peripheral Optic Radii (Zonal Curvatures) for the following:
BCOR 7.0 to 8.8 in 0.1 steps
Zone Width 0.4   Zone Inner Diameters 7.0 to 10.4 in 0.2 steps
Axial Edge Lift Components 0.01 to 0.15 in 0.01 steps

```
FOR EDGE LIFT   0.01 ,   OPTIC DIAMETERS   7  -  7.8 ,    ZONAL CURVATURES ARE
 7.2  7.3  7.45  7.55  7.65  7.75  7.85  8  8.1  8.2  8.3  8.45  8.55  8.65  8.75  8.9  9  9.1  9.2

FOR EDGE LIFT   0.01 ,   OPTIC DIAMETERS   7.2  -  8 ,    ZONAL CURVATURES ARE
 7.2  7.3  7.4  7.55  7.65  7.75  7.85  7.95  8.1  8.2  8.3  8.4  8.5  8.65  8.75  8.85  8.95  9.1  9.2

FOR EDGE LIFT   0.01 ,   OPTIC DIAMETERS   7.4  -  8.2 ,    ZONAL CURVATURES ARE
 7.2  7.3  7.4  7.5  7.65  7.75  7.85  7.95  8.05  8.2  8.3  8.4  8.5  8.6  8.75  8.85  8.95  9.05  9.2

FOR EDGE LIFT   0.01 ,   OPTIC DIAMETERS   7.6  -  8.4 ,    ZONAL CURVATURES ARE
 7.2  7.3  7.4  7.5  7.6  7.7  7.85  7.95  8.05  8.15  8.25  8.4  8.5  8.6  8.7  8.85  8.95  9.05  9.15

FOR EDGE LIFT   0.01 ,   OPTIC DIAMETERS   7.8  -  8.6 ,    ZONAL CURVATURES ARE
 7.15  7.25  7.4  7.5  7.6  7.7  7.8  7.95  8.05  8.15  8.25  8.35  8.5  8.6  8.7  8.8  8.9  9.05  9.15

FOR EDGE LIFT   0.01 ,   OPTIC DIAMETERS   8.  -  8.8 ,    ZONAL CURVATURES ARE
 7.15  7.25  7.35  7.5  7.6  7.7  7.8  7.9  8.05  8.15  8.25  8.35  8.45  8.6  8.7  8.8  8.9  9  9.15

FOR EDGE LIFT   0.01 ,   OPTIC DIAMETERS   8.2  -  9. ,    ZONAL CURVATURES ARE
 7.15  7.25  7.35  7.45  7.6  7.7  7.8  7.9  8  8.1  8.25  8.35  8.45  8.55  8.65  8.8  8.9  9  9.1

FOR EDGE LIFT   0.01 ,   OPTIC DIAMETERS   8.4  -  9.2 ,    ZONAL CURVATURES ARE
 7.15  7.25  7.35  7.45  7.55  7.7  7.8  7.9  8  8.1  8.2  8.35  8.45  8.55  8.65  8.75  8.9  9  9.1
```

```
FOR EDGE LIFT   0.01 ,   OPTIC DIAMETERS   8.6  -  9.4 ,    ZONAL CURVATURES ARE
 7.15  7.25  7.35  7.45  7.55  7.65  7.75  7.9  8  8.1  8.2  8.3  8.45  8.55  8.65  8.75  8.85  9  9.1

FOR EDGE LIFT   0.01 ,   OPTIC DIAMETERS   8.8  -  9.6 ,    ZONAL CURVATURES ARE
 7.1  7.2  7.35  7.45  7.55  7.65  7.75  7.85  8  8.1  8.2  8.3  8.4  8.55  8.65  8.75  8.85  8.95  9.05

FOR EDGE LIFT   0.01 ,   OPTIC DIAMETERS   9.  -  9.8 ,    ZONAL CURVATURES ARE
 7.1  7.2  7.3  7.45  7.55  7.65  7.75  7.85  7.95  8.1  8.2  8.3  8.4  8.5  8.6  8.75  8.85  8.95  9.05

FOR EDGE LIFT   0.01 ,   OPTIC DIAMETERS   9.2  -  10. ,    ZONAL CURVATURES ARE
 7.1  7.2  7.3  7.4  7.55  7.65  7.75  7.85  7.95  8.05  8.2  8.3  8.4  8.5  8.6  8.7  8.85  8.95  9.05

FOR EDGE LIFT   0.01 ,   OPTIC DIAMETERS   9.4  -  10.2 ,    ZONAL CURVATURES ARE
 7.1  7.2  7.3  7.4  7.5  7.65  7.75  7.85  7.95  8.05  8.15  8.3  8.4  8.5  8.6  8.7  8.8  8.95  9.05

FOR EDGE LIFT   0.01 ,   OPTIC DIAMETERS   9.6  -  10.4 ,    ZONAL CURVATURES ARE
 7.1  7.2  7.3  7.4  7.5  7.6  7.75  7.85  7.95  8.05  8.15  8.25  8.35  8.5  8.6  8.7  8.8  8.9  9

FOR EDGE LIFT   0.01 ,   OPTIC DIAMETERS   9.8  -  10.6 ,    ZONAL CURVATURES ARE
 7.1  7.2  7.3  7.4  7.5  7.6  7.7  7.85  7.95  8.05  8.15  8.25  8.35  8.45  8.6  8.7  8.8  8.9  9

FOR EDGE LIFT   0.01 ,   OPTIC DIAMETERS   10.  -  10.8 ,    ZONAL CURVATURES ARE
 7.05  7.2  7.3  7.4  7.5  7.6  7.7  7.8  7.9  8.05  8.15  8.25  8.35  8.45  8.55  8.7  8.8  8.9  9

FOR EDGE LIFT   0.01 ,   OPTIC DIAMETERS   10.2  -  11. ,    ZONAL CURVATURES ARE
 7.05  7.15  7.3  7.4  7.5  7.6  7.7  7.8  7.9  8  8.15  8.25  8.35  8.45  8.55  8.65  8.8  8.9  9

FOR EDGE LIFT   0.01 ,   OPTIC DIAMETERS   1C.4  -  11.2 ,    ZONAL CURVATURES ARE
 7.05  7.15  7.25  7.4  7.5  7.6  7.7  7.8  7.9  8  8.1  8.25  8.35  8.45  8.55  8.65  8.75  8.9  9
```

```
FOR EDGE LIFT   0.02 ,   OPTIC DIAMETERS   7  -  7.8 ,   ZONAL CURVATURES ARE
 7.45  7.55  7.7  7.8  7.95  8.05  8.2  8.3  8.4  8.55  8.65  8.8  8.9  9.05  9.15  9.3  9.45  9.55  9.7

FOR EDGE LIFT   0.02 ,   OPTIC DIAMETERS   7.2  -  8 ,   ZONAL CURVATURES ARE
 7.4  7.55  7.65  7.8  7.9  8  8.15  8.25  8.4  8.5  8.65  8.75  8.9  9  9.15  9.25  9.4  9.5  9.65

FOR EDGE LIFT   0.02 ,   OPTIC DIAMETERS   7.4  -  8.2 ,   ZONAL CURVATURES ARE
 7.4  7.5  7.65  7.75  7.85  8  8.1  8.25  8.35  8.5  8.6  8.75  8.85  9  9.1  9.25  9.35  9.5  9.6

FOR EDGE LIFT   0.02 ,   OPTIC DIAMETERS   7.6  -  8.4 ,   ZONAL CURVATURES ARE
 7.35  7.5  7.6  7.75  7.85  7.95  8.1  8.2  8.35  8.45  8.55  8.7  8.8  8.95  9.05  9.2  9.3  9.45  9.55

FOR EDGE LIFT   0.02 ,   OPTIC DIAMETERS   7.8  -  8.6 ,   ZONAL CURVATURES ARE
 7.35  7.45  7.6  7.7  7.8  7.95  8.05  8.2  8.3  8.4  8.55  8.65  8.8  8.9  9.05  9.15  9.3  9.4  9.55

FOR EDGE LIFT   0.02 ,   OPTIC DIAMETERS   8.  -  8.8 ,   ZONAL CURVATURES ARE
 7.3  7.45  7.55  7.7  7.8  7.9  8.05  8.15  8.25  8.4  8.5  8.65  8.75  8.9  9  9.15  9.25  9.35  9.5

FOR EDGE LIFT   0.02 ,   OPTIC DIAMETERS   8.2  -  9. ,   ZONAL CURVATURES ARE
 7.3  7.4  7.55  7.65  7.75  7.9  8  8.15  8.25  8.35  8.5  8.6  8.75  8.85  8.95  9.1  9.2  9.35  9.45

FOR EDGE LIFT   0.02 ,   OPTIC DIAMETERS   8.4  -  9.2 ,   ZONAL CURVATURES ARE
 7.3  7.4  7.5  7.65  7.75  7.85  8  8.1  8.2  8.35  8.45  8.6  8.7  8.8  8.95  9.05  9.2  9.3  9.45

FOR EDGE LIFT   0.02 ,   OPTIC DIAMETERS   8.6  -  9.4 ,   ZONAL CURVATURES ARE
 7.25  7.4  7.5  7.6  7.75  7.85  7.95  8.1  8.2  8.3  8.45  8.55  8.7  8.8  8.9  9.05  9.15  9.3  9.4
```

```
FOR EDGE LIFT   0.02 ,   OPTIC DIAMETERS   8.8  -  9.6 ,    ZONAL CURVATURES ARE
 7.25  7.35  7.5  7.6  7.7  7.8  7.95  8.05  8.2  8.3  8.4  8.55  8.65  8.75  8.9  9  9.15  9.25  9.35

FOR EDGE LIFT   0.02 ,   OPTIC DIAMETERS   9.  -  9.8 ,    ZONAL CURVATURES ARE
 7.25  7.35  7.45  7.55  7.7  7.8  7.9  8.05  8.15  8.25  8.4  8.5  8.65  8.75  8.85  9  9.1  9.25  9.35

FOR EDGE LIFT   0.02 ,   OPTIC DIAMETERS   9.2  -  10. ,    ZONAL CURVATURES ARE
 7.2  7.3  7.45  7.55  7.65  7.8  7.9  8  8.15  8.25  8.35  8.5  8.6  8.7  8.85  8.95  9.1  9.2  9.3

FOR EDGE LIFT   0.02 ,   OPTIC DIAMETERS   9.4  -  10.2 ,    ZONAL CURVATURES ARE
 7.2  7.3  7.4  7.55  7.65  7.75  7.9  8  8.1  8.25  8.35  8.45  8.6  8.7  8.8  8.95  9.05  9.15  9.3

FOR EDGE LIFT   0.02 ,   OPTIC DIAMETERS   9.6  -  10.4 ,    ZONAL CURVATURES ARE
 7.2  7.3  7.4  7.5  7.65  7.75  7.85  8  8.1  8.2  8.35  8.45  8.55  8.7  8.8  8.9  9.05  9.15  9.25

FOR EDGE LIFT   0.02 ,   OPTIC DIAMETERS   9.8  -  10.6 ,    ZONAL CURVATURES ARE
 7.15  7.3  7.4  7.5  7.6  7.75  7.85  7.95  8.1  8.2  8.3  8.4  8.55  8.65  8.75  8.9  9  9.15  9.25

FOR EDGE LIFT   0.02 ,   OPTIC DIAMETERS   10.  -  10.8 ,    ZONAL CURVATURES ARE
 7.15  7.25  7.35  7.5  7.6  7.7  7.85  7.95  8.05  8.15  8.3  8.4  8.5  8.65  8.75  8.85  9  9.1  9.2

FOR EDGE LIFT   0.02 ,   OPTIC DIAMETERS   10.2  -  11. ,    ZONAL CURVATURES ARE
 7.15  7.25  7.35  7.45  7.6  7.7  7.8  7.95  8.05  8.15  8.25  8.4  8.5  8.6  8.75  8.85  8.95  9.1  9.2

FOR EDGE LIFT   0.02 ,   OPTIC DIAMETERS   10.4  -  11.2 ,    ZONAL CURVATURES ARE
 7.1  7.25  7.35  7.45  7.55  7.7  7.8  7.9  8.05  8.15  8.25  8.35  8.5  8.6  8.7  8.85  8.95  9.05  9.2
```

```
FOR EDGE LIFT   0.03 ,   OPTIC DIAMETERS   7  -  7.8 ,    ZONAL CURVATURES ARE
 7.7  7.85  7.95  8.1  8.25  8.4  8.5  8.65  8.8  8.95  9.05  9.2  9.35  9.5  9.65  9.8  9.95  10.05  10.2

FOR EDGE LIFT   0.03 ,   OPTIC DIAMETERS   7.2  -  8 ,    ZONAL CURVATURES ARE
 7.65  7.8  7.9  8.05  8.2  8.35  8.45  8.6  8.75  8.9  9  9.15  9.3  9.45  9.6  9.7  9.85  10  10.15

FOR EDGE LIFT   0.03 ,   OPTIC DIAMETERS   7.4  -  8.2 ,    ZONAL CURVATURES ARE
 7.6  7.75  7.9  8  8.15  8.3  8.4  8.55  8.7  8.8  8.95  9.1  9.25  9.4  9.5  9.65  9.8  9.95  10.1

FOR EDGE LIFT   0.03 ,   OPTIC DIAMETERS   7.6  -  8.4 ,    ZONAL CURVATURES ARE
 7.6  7.7  7.85  7.95  8.1  8.25  8.35  8.5  8.65  8.75  8.9  9.05  9.2  9.3  9.45  9.6  9.75  9.9  10

FOR EDGE LIFT   0.03 ,   OPTIC DIAMETERS   7.8  -  8.6 ,    ZONAL CURVATURES ARE
 7.55  7.65  7.8  7.95  8.05  8.2  8.35  8.45  8.6  8.75  8.85  9  9.15  9.25  9.4  9.55  9.7  9.8  9.95

FOR EDGE LIFT   0.03 ,   OPTIC DIAMETERS   8.  -  8.8 ,    ZONAL CURVATURES ARE
 7.5  7.65  7.75  7.9  8  8.15  8.3  8.4  8.55  8.7  8.8  8.95  9.1  9.2  9.35  9.5  9.65  9.75  9.9

FOR EDGE LIFT   0.03 ,   OPTIC DIAMETERS   8.2  -  9. ,    ZONAL CURVATURES ARE
 7.45  7.6  7.75  7.85  8  8.1  8.25  8.35  8.5  8.65  8.75  8.9  9.05  9.15  9.3  9.45  9.6  9.7  9.85

FOR EDGE LIFT   0.03 ,   OPTIC DIAMETERS   8.4  -  9.2 ,    ZONAL CURVATURES ARE
 7.45  7.55  7.7  7.8  7.95  8.1  8.2  8.35  8.45  8.6  8.75  8.85  9  9.15  9.25  9.4  9.55  9.65  9.8

FOR EDGE LIFT   0.03 ,   OPTIC DIAMETERS   8.6  -  9.4 ,    ZONAL CURVATURES ARE
 7.4  7.55  7.65  7.8  7.9  8.05  8.15  8.3  8.45  8.55  8.7  8.8  8.95  9.1  9.2  9.35  9.5  9.6  9.75
```

```
FOR EDGE LIFT   0.03 ,   OPTIC DIAMETERS   8.8  -  9.6 ,    ZONAL CURVATURES ARE
 7.4  7.5  7.65  7.75  7.9  8  8.15  8.25  8.4  8.5  8.65  8.8  8.9  9.05  9.15  9.3  9.45  9.55  9.7

FOR EDGE LIFT   0.03 ,   OPTIC DIAMETERS   9.  -  9.8 ,    ZONAL CURVATURES ARE
 7.35  7.5  7.6  7.7  7.85  8  8.1  8.25  8.35  8.5  8.6  8.75  8.85  9  9.15  9.25  9.4  9.55  9.65

FOR EDGE LIFT   0.03 ,   OPTIC DIAMETERS   9.2  -  10. ,    ZONAL CURVATURES ARE
 7.35  7.45  7.55  7.7  7.8  7.95  8.05  8.2  8.3  8.45  8.6  8.7  8.85  8.95  9.1  9.2  9.35  9.5  9.6

FOR EDGE LIFT   0.03 ,   OPTIC DIAMETERS   9.4  -  10.2 ,    ZONAL CURVATURES ARE
 7.3  7.4  7.55  7.65  7.8  7.9  8.05  8.15  8.3  8.4  8.55  8.65  8.8  8.95  9.05  9.2  9.3  9.45  9.6

FOR EDGE LIFT   0.03 ,   OPTIC DIAMETERS   9.6  -  10.4 ,    ZONAL CURVATURES ARE
 7.3  7.4  7.5  7.65  7.75  7.9  8  8.15  8.25  8.4  8.5  8.65  8.75  8.9  9  9.15  9.3  9.4  9.55

FOR EDGE LIFT   0.03 ,   OPTIC DIAMETERS   9.8  -  10.6 ,    ZONAL CURVATURES ARE
 7.25  7.35  7.5  7.6  7.75  7.85  8  8.1  8.25  8.35  8.5  8.6  8.75  8.85  9  9.1  9.25  9.35  9.5

FOR EDGE LIFT   0.03 ,   OPTIC DIAMETERS   10.  -  10.8 ,    ZONAL CURVATURES ARE
 7.25  7.35  7.45  7.6  7.7  7.85  7.95  8.1  8.2  8.35  8.45  8.6  8.7  8.85  8.95  9.1  9.2  9.35  9.45

FOR EDGE LIFT   0.03 ,   OPTIC DIAMETERS   10.2  -  11. ,    ZONAL CURVATURES ARE
 7.2  7.35  7.45  7.55  7.7  7.8  7.95  8.05  8.2  8.3  8.4  8.55  8.65  8.8  8.9  9.05  9.15  9.3  9.45

FOR EDGE LIFT   0.03 ,   OPTIC DIAMETERS   10.4  -  11.2 ,    ZONAL CURVATURES ARE
 7.2  7.3  7.45  7.55  7.65  7.8  7.9  8.05  8.15  8.25  8.4  8.5  8.65  8.75  8.9  9  9.15  9.25  9.4
```

```
FOR EDGE LIFT   0.04 ,   OPTIC DIAMETERS   7  -  7.8 ,    ZONAL CURVATURES ARE
 8  8.15  8.3  8.45  8.6  8.75  8.9  9.05  9.2  9.35  9.5  9.7  9.85  10  10.15  10.35  10.5  10.65  10.85

FOR EDGE LIFT   0.04 ,   OPTIC DIAMETERS   7.2  -  8 ,    ZONAL CURVATURES ARE
 7.9  8.05  8.2  8.35  8.5  8.65  8.8  8.95  9.15  9.3  9.45  9.6  9.75  9.9  10.05  10.25  10.4  10.55  10.75

FOR EDGE LIFT   0.04 ,   OPTIC DIAMETERS   7.4  -  8.2 ,    ZONAL CURVATURES ARE
 7.85  8  8.15  8.3  8.45  8.6  8.75  8.9  9.05  9.2  9.35  9.5  9.65  9.85  10  10.15  10.3  10.45  10.65

FOR EDGE LIFT   0.04 ,   OPTIC DIAMETERS   7.6  -  8.4 ,    ZONAL CURVATURES ARE
 7.8  7.95  8.1  8.25  8.4  8.55  8.7  8.85  9  9.15  9.3  9.45  9.6  9.75  9.9  10.05  10.2  10.35  10.55

FOR EDGE LIFT   0.04 ,   OPTIC DIAMETERS   7.8  -  8.6 ,    ZONAL CURVATURES ARE
 7.75  7.9  8.05  8.2  8.35  8.45  8.6  8.75  8.9  9.05  9.2  9.35  9.5  9.65  9.8  10  10.15  10.3  10.45

FOR EDGE LIFT   0.04 ,   OPTIC DIAMETERS   8.  -  8.8 ,    ZONAL CURVATURES ARE
 7.7  7.85  8  8.15  8.25  8.4  8.55  8.7  8.85  9  9.15  9.3  9.45  9.6  9.75  9.9  10.05  10.2  10.35

FOR EDGE LIFT   0.04 ,   OPTIC DIAMETERS   8.2  -  9. ,    ZONAL CURVATURES ARE
 7.65  7.8  7.95  8.05  8.2  8.35  8.5  8.65  8.8  8.95  9.1  9.25  9.4  9.55  9.7  9.85  10  10.15  10.3

FOR EDGE LIFT   0.04 ,   OPTIC DIAMETERS   8.4  -  9.2 ,    ZONAL CURVATURES ARE
 7.6  7.75  7.9  8  8.15  8.3  8.45  8.6  8.75  8.9  9  9.15  9.3  9.45  9.6  9.75  9.9  10.05  10.2

FOR EDGE LIFT   0.04 ,   OPTIC DIAMETERS   8.6  -  9.4 ,    ZONAL CURVATURES ARE
 7.55  7.7  7.85  8  8.1  8.25  8.4  8.55  8.7  8.8  8.95  9.1  9.25  9.4  9.55  9.7  9.85  10  10.15
```

FOR EDGE LIFT 0.04 , OPTIC DIAMETERS 8.8 - 9.6 , ZONAL CURVATURES ARE

7.55 7.65 7.8 7.95 8.05 8.2 8.35 8.5 8.65 8.75 8.9 9.05 9.2 9.35 9.5 9.65 9.8 9.9 10.05

FOR EDGE LIFT 0.04 , OPTIC DIAMETERS 9. - 9.8 , ZONAL CURVATURES ARE

7.5 7.6 7.75 7.9 8 8.15 8.3 8.45 8.6 8.7 8.85 9 9.15 9.3 9.45 9.55 9.7 9.85 10

FOR EDGE LIFT 0.04 , OPTIC DIAMETERS 9.2 - 10. , ZONAL CURVATURES ARE

7.45 7.6 7.7 7.85 8 8.1 8.25 8.4 8.55 8.65 8.3 8.95 9.1 9.25 9.35 9.5 9.65 9.8 9.95

FOR EDGE LIFT 0.04 , OPTIC DIAMETERS 9.4 - 10.2 , ZONAL CURVATURES ARE

7.4 7.55 7.7 7.8 7.95 8.1 8.2 8.35 8.5 8.6 8.75 8.9 9.05 9.2 9.3 9.45 9.6 9.75 9.9

FOR EDGE LIFT 0.04 , OPTIC DIAMETERS 9.6 - 10.4 , ZONAL CURVATURES ARE

7.4 7.5 7.65 7.75 7.9 8.05 8.15 8.3 8.45 8.55 8.7 8.85 9 9.15 9.25 9.4 9.55 9.7 9.85

FOR EDGE LIFT 0.04 , OPTIC DIAMETERS 9.8 - 10.6 , ZONAL CURVATURES ARE

7.35 7.5 7.6 7.75 7.85 8 8.15 8.25 8.4 8.55 8.65 8.8 8.95 9.1 9.2 9.35 9.5 9.65 9.8

FOR EDGE LIFT 0.04 , OPTIC DIAMETERS 10. - 10.8 , ZONAL CURVATURES ARE

7.3 7.45 7.55 7.7 7.85 7.95 8.1 8.2 8.35 8.5 8.65 8.75 8.9 9.05 9.15 9.3 9.45 9.6 9.75

FOR EDGE LIFT 0.04 , OPTIC DIAMETERS 10.2 - 11. , ZONAL CURVATURES ARE

7.3 7.4 7.55 7.65 7.8 7.95 8.05 8.2 8.3 8.45 8.6 8.7 8.85 9 9.1 9.25 9.4 9.55 9.7

FOR EDGE LIFT 0.04 , OPTIC DIAMETERS 10.4 - 11.2 , ZONAL CURVATURES ARE

7.25 7.4 7.5 7.65 7.75 7.9 8 8.15 8.3 8.4 8.55 8.7 8.8 8.95 9.1 9.2 9.35 9.5 9.65

```
FOR EDGE LIFT   0.05 ,   OPTIC DIAMETERS   7  -  7.8 ,    ZONAL CURVATURES ARE
 8.3  8.45  8.65  8.8  8.95  9.15  9.3  9.5  9.65  9.85  10.05  10.2  10.4  10.6  10.75  10.95  11.15  11.35  11.55

FOR EDGE LIFT   0.05 ,   OPTIC DIAMETERS   7.2  -  8 ,    ZONAL CURVATURES ARE
 8.2  8.4  8.55  8.7  8.9  9.05  9.2  9.4  9.55  9.75  9.9  10.1  10.25  10.45  10.65  10.8  11  11.2  11.4

FOR EDGE LIFT   0.05 ,   OPTIC DIAMETERS   7.4  -  8.2 ,    ZONAL CURVATURES ARE
 8.15  8.3  8.45  8.6  8.8  8.95  9.1  9.3  9.45  9.65  9.8  10  10.15  10.35  10.5  10.7  10.9  11.05  11.25

FOR EDGE LIFT   0.05 ,   OPTIC DIAMETERS   7.6  -  8.4 ,    ZONAL CURVATURES ARE
 8.05  8.2  8.4  8.55  8.7  8.85  9.05  9.2  9.35  9.55  9.7  9.85  10.05  10.2  10.4  10.6  10.75  10.95  11.1

FOR EDGE LIFT   0.05 ,   OPTIC DIAMETERS   7.8  -  8.6 ,    ZONAL CURVATURES ARE
 8  8.15  8.3  8.45  8.6  8.8  8.95  9.1  9.25  9.45  9.6  9.75  9.95  10.1  10.3  10.45  10.65  10.8  11

FOR EDGE LIFT   0.05 ,   OPTIC DIAMETERS   8.  -  8.8 ,    ZONAL CURVATURES ARE
 7.9  8.05  8.25  8.4  8.55  8.7  8.85  9  9.2  9.35  9.5  9.7  9.85  10  10.2  10.35  10.55  10.7  10.9

FOR EDGE LIFT   0.05 ,   OPTIC DIAMETERS   8.2  -  9. ,    ZONAL CURVATURES ARE
 7.85  8  8.15  8.3  8.45  8.65  8.8  8.95  9.1  9.25  9.45  9.6  9.75  9.9  10.1  10.25  10.45  10.6  10.8

FOR EDGE LIFT   0.05 ,   OPTIC DIAMETERS   8.4  -  9.2 ,    ZONAL CURVATURES ARE
 7.8  7.95  8.1  8.25  8.4  8.55  8.7  8.85  9  9.2  9.35  9.5  9.65  9.85  10  10.15  10.35  10.5  10.65

FOR EDGE LIFT   0.05 ,   OPTIC DIAMETERS   8.6  -  9.4 ,    ZONAL CURVATURES ARE
 7.75  7.9  8.05  8.2  8.35  8.5  8.65  8.8  8.95  9.1  9.25  9.45  9.6  9.75  9.9  10.05  10.25  10.4  10.6
```

```
FOR EDGE LIFT   0.05 ,   OPTIC DIAMETERS   8.8  -  9.6 ,    ZONAL CURVATURES ARE
 7.7  7.85  8  8.1  8.25  8.4  8.55  8.75  8.9  9.05  9.2  9.35  9.5  9.65  9.85  10  10.15  10.3  10.5

FOR EDGE LIFT   0.05 ,   OPTIC DIAMETERS   9.  -  9.8 ,    ZONAL CURVATURES ARE
 7.65  7.8  7.9  8.05  8.2  8.35  8.5  8.65  8.8  8.95  9.1  9.3  9.45  9.6  9.75  9.9  10.05  10.25  10.4

FOR EDGE LIFT   0.05 ,   OPTIC DIAMETERS   9.2  -  10. ,    ZONAL CURVATURES ARE
 7.6  7.75  7.85  8  8.15  8.3  8.45  8.6  8.75  8.9  9.05  9.2  9.35  9.5  9.65  9.85  10  10.15  10.3

FOR EDGE LIFT   0.05 ,   OPTIC DIAMETERS   9.4  -  10.2 ,    ZONAL CURVATURES ARE
 7.55  7.7  7.8  7.95  8.1  8.25  8.4  8.55  8.7  8.85  9  9.15  9.3  9.45  9.6  9.75  9.9  10.05  10.25

FOR EDGE LIFT   0.05 ,   OPTIC DIAMETERS   9.6  -  10.4 ,    ZONAL CURVATURES ARE
 7.5  7.65  7.75  7.9  8.05  8.2  8.35  8.5  8.65  8.8  8.95  9.1  9.25  9.4  9.55  9.7  9.85  10  10.15

FOR EDGE LIFT   0.05 ,   OPTIC DIAMETERS   9.8  -  10.6 ,    ZONAL CURVATURES ARE
 7.45  7.6  7.7  7.85  8  8.15  8.3  8.45  8.6  8.7  8.85  9  9.15  9.3  9.45  9.6  9.75  9.95  10.1

FOR EDGE LIFT   0.05 ,   OPTIC DIAMETERS   10.  -  10.8 ,    ZONAL CURVATURES ARE
 7.4  7.55  7.7  7.8  7.95  8.1  8.25  8.4  8.5  8.65  8.8  8.95  9.1  9.25  9.4  9.55  9.7  9.85  10

FOR EDGE LIFT   0.05 ,   OPTIC DIAMETERS   10.2  -  11. ,    ZONAL CURVATURES ARE
 7.35  7.5  7.65  7.8  7.9  8.05  8.2  8.35  8.45  8.6  8.75  8.9  9.05  9.2  9.35  9.5  9.65  9.8  9.95

FOR EDGE LIFT   0.05 ,   OPTIC DIAMETERS   10.4  -  11.2 ,    ZONAL CURVATURES ARE
 7.35  7.45  7.6  7.75  7.85  8  8.15  8.3  8.45  8.55  8.7  8.85  9  9.15  9.3  9.45  9.6  9.75  9.9
```

```
FOR EDGE LIFT   6.00000E-2 ,   OPTIC DIAMETERS   7 - 7.8 ,   ZONAL CURVATURES ARE
 8.65  8.85  9.05  9.2  9.4  9.6  9.8  10  10.2  10.4  10.6  10.85  11.05  11.25  11.45  11.7  11.9  12.15  12.35

FOR EDGE LIFT   6.00000E-2 ,   OPTIC DIAMETERS   7.2 - 8 ,   ZONAL CURVATURES ARE
 8.55  8.7  8.9  9.1  9.3  9.45  9.65  9.85  10.05  10.25  10.45  10.65  10.85  11.1  11.3  11.5  11.7  11.95  12.15

FOR EDGE LIFT   6.00000E-2 ,   OPTIC DIAMETERS   7.4 - 8.2 ,   ZONAL CURVATURES ARE
 8.45  8.6  8.8  9  9.15  9.35  9.55  9.75  9.9  10.1  10.3  10.5  10.7  10.9  11.1  11.35  11.55  11.75  11.95

FOR EDGE LIFT   6.00000E-2 ,   OPTIC DIAMETERS   7.6 - 8.4 ,   ZONAL CURVATURES ARE
 8.35  8.5  8.7  8.85  9.05  9.25  9.4  9.6  9.8  10  10.15  10.35  10.55  10.75  10.95  11.15  11.4  11.6  11.8

FOR EDGE LIFT   6.00000E-2 ,   OPTIC DIAMETERS   7.8 - 8.6 ,   ZONAL CURVATURES ARE
 8.25  8.4  8.6  8.75  8.95  9.1  9.3  9.5  9.65  9.85  10.05  10.25  10.45  10.6  10.8  11  11.2  11.4  11.65

FOR EDGE LIFT   6.00000E-2 ,   OPTIC DIAMETERS   8. - 8.8 ,   ZONAL CURVATURES ARE
 8.15  8.35  8.5  8.65  8.85  9  9.2  9.4  9.55  9.75  9.9  10.1  10.3  10.5  10.7  10.9  11.1  11.25  11.5

FOR EDGE LIFT   6.00000E-2 ,   OPTIC DIAMETERS   8.2 - 9. ,   ZONAL CURVATURES ARE
 8.1  8.25  8.4  8.6  8.75  8.9  9.1  9.25  9.45  9.65  9.8  10  10.2  10.35  10.55  10.75  10.95  11.15  11.35

FOR EDGE LIFT   6.00000E-2 ,   OPTIC DIAMETERS   8.4 - 9.2 ,   ZONAL CURVATURES ARE
 8  8.15  8.35  8.5  8.65  8.85  9  9.15  9.35  9.5  9.7  9.9  10.05  10.25  10.45  10.6  10.8  11  11.2

FOR EDGE LIFT   6.00000E-2 ,   OPTIC DIAMETERS   8.6 - 9.4 ,   ZONAL CURVATURES ARE
 7.95  8.1  8.25  8.4  8.6  8.75  8.9  9.1  9.25  9.45  9.6  9.8  9.95  10.15  10.3  10.5  10.7  10.85  11.05
```

```
FOR EDGE LIFT   6.00000E-2 ,   OPTIC DIAMETERS   8.8  -  9.6 ,    ZONAL CURVATURES ARE
 7.85  8  8.15  8.35  8.5  8.65  8.85  9  9.15  9.35  9.5  9.7  9.85  10.05  10.2  10.4  10.55  10.75  10.95

FOR EDGE LIFT   6.00000E-2 ,   OPTIC DIAMETERS   9.  -  9.8 ,    ZONAL CURVATURES ARE
 7.8  7.95  8.1  8.25  8.4  8.6  8.75  8.9  9.1  9.25  9.4  9.6  9.75  9.95  10.1  10.3  10.45  10.65  10.85

FOR EDGE LIFT   6.00000E-2 ,   OPTIC DIAMETERS   9.2  -  10. ,    ZONAL CURVATURES ARE
 7.75  7.9  8.05  8.2  8.35  8.5  8.65  8.85  9  9.15  9.35  9.5  9.65  9.85  10  10.2  10.35  10.55  10.7

FOR EDGE LIFT   6.00000E-2 ,   OPTIC DIAMETERS   9.4  -  10.2 ,    ZONAL CURVATURES ARE
 7.65  7.8  7.95  8.1  8.3  8.45  8.6  8.75  8.9  9.1  9.25  9.4  9.6  9.75  9.9  10.1  10.25  10.45  10.6

FOR EDGE LIFT   6.00000E-2 ,   OPTIC DIAMETERS   9.6  -  10.4 ,    ZONAL CURVATURES ARE
 7.6  7.75  7.9  8.05  8.2  8.35  8.55  8.7  8.85  9  9.15  9.35  9.5  9.65  9.85  10  10.15  10.35  10.5

FOR EDGE LIFT   6.00000E-2 ,   OPTIC DIAMETERS   9.8  -  10.6 ,    ZONAL CURVATURES ARE
 7.55  7.7  7.85  8  8.15  8.3  8.45  8.6  8.75  8.95  9.1  9.25  9.4  9.6  9.75  9.9  10.1  10.25  10.4

FOR EDGE LIFT   6.00000E-2 ,   OPTIC DIAMETERS   10.  -  10.8 ,    ZONAL CURVATURES ARE
 7.5  7.65  7.8  7.95  8.1  8.25  8.4  8.55  8.7  8.85  9  9.2  9.35  9.5  9.65  9.85  10  10.15  10.35

FOR EDGE LIFT   6.00000E-2 ,   OPTIC DIAMETERS   10.2  -  11. ,    ZONAL CURVATURES ARE
 7.45  7.6  7.75  7.9  8.05  8.2  8.35  8.5  8.65  8.8  8.95  9.1  9.25  9.4  9.6  9.75  9.9  10.1  10.25

FOR EDGE LIFT   6.00000E-2 ,   OPTIC DIAMETERS   10.4  -  11.2 ,    ZONAL CURVATURES ARE
 7.4  7.55  7.7  7.85  8  8.15  8.3  8.45  8.6  8.75  8.9  9.05  9.2  9.35  9.5  9.65  9.85  10  10.15
```

```
FOR EDGE LIFT   0.07 ,   OPTIC DIAMETERS   7  -  7.8 ,    ZONAL CURVATURES ARE
 9.05  9.25  9.45  9.7  9.9  10.15  10.35  10.6  10.8  11.05  11.3  11.55  11.8  12.05  12.3  12.55  12.8  13.05  13.35

FOR EDGE LIFT   0.07 ,   OPTIC DIAMETERS   7.2  -  8 ,    ZONAL CURVATURES ARE
 8.9  9.1  9.3  9.55  9.75  9.95  10.15  10.4  10.6  10.85  11.1  11.3  11.55  11.8  12.05  12.3  12.55  12.8  13.05

FOR EDGE LIFT   0.07 ,   OPTIC DIAMETERS   7.4  -  8.2 ,    ZONAL CURVATURES ARE
 8.75  8.95  9.15  9.4  9.6  9.8  10  10.2  10.45  10.65  10.9  11.1  11.35  11.6  11.8  12.05  12.3  12.55  12.8

FOR EDGE LIFT   0.07 ,   OPTIC DIAMETERS   7.6  -  8.4 ,    ZONAL CURVATURES ARE
 8.65  8.85  9.05  9.25  9.45  9.65  9.85  10.05  10.3  10.5  10.7  10.95  11.15  11.4  11.6  11.85  12.1  12.35  12.6

FOR EDGE LIFT   0.07 ,   OPTIC DIAMETERS   7.8  -  8.6 ,    ZONAL CURVATURES ARE
 8.55  8.7  8.9  9.1  9.3  9.5  9.7  9.9  10.1  10.35  10.55  10.75  11  11.2  11.45  11.65  11.9  12.1  12.35

FOR EDGE LIFT   0.07 ,   OPTIC DIAMETERS   8.  -  8.8 ,    ZONAL CURVATURES ARE
 8.4  8.6  8.8  9  9.2  9.35  9.55  9.75  9.95  10.2  10.4  10.6  10.8  11.05  11.25  11.45  11.7  11.9  12.15

FOR EDGE LIFT   0.07 ,   OPTIC DIAMETERS   8.2  -  9. ,    ZONAL CURVATURES ARE
 8.3  8.5  8.7  8.85  9.05  9.25  9.45  9.65  9.85  10.05  10.25  10.45  10.65  10.85  11.1  11.3  11.5  11.75  11.95

FOR EDGE LIFT   0.07 ,   OPTIC DIAMETERS   8.4  -  9.2 ,    ZONAL CURVATURES ARE
 8.2  8.4  8.6  8.75  8.95  9.15  9.3  9.5  9.7  9.9  10.1  10.3  10.5  10.7  10.9  11.15  11.35  11.55  11.8

FOR EDGE LIFT   0.07 ,   OPTIC DIAMETERS   8.6  -  9.4 ,    ZONAL CURVATURES ARE
 8.15  8.3  8.5  8.65  8.85  9  9.2  9.4  9.6  9.8  9.95  10.15  10.35  10.55  10.75  11  11.2  11.4  11.6
```

```
FOR EDGE LIFT   0.07 ,   OPTIC DIAMETERS   8.8  -  9.6 ,   ZONAL CURVATURES ARE
 8.05  8.2  8.4  8.55  8.75  8.9  9.1  9.3  9.45  9.65  9.85  10.05  10.25  10.45  10.65  10.85  11.05  11.25  11.45

FOR EDGE LIFT   0.07 ,   OPTIC DIAMETERS   9.  -  9.8 ,   ZONAL CURVATURES ARE
 7.95  8.15  8.3  8.45  8.65  8.8  9  9.2  9.35  9.55  9.75  9.9  10.1  10.3  10.5  10.7  10.9  11.1  11.3

FOR EDGE LIFT   0.07 ,   OPTIC DIAMETERS   9.2  -  10. ,   ZONAL CURVATURES ARE
 7.9  8.05  8.2  8.4  8.55  8.75  8.9  9.1  9.25  9.45  9.65  9.8  10  10.2  10.4  10.55  10.75  10.95  11.15

FOR EDGE LIFT   0.07 ,   OPTIC DIAMETERS   9.4  -  10.2 ,   ZONAL CURVATURES ARE
 7.8  7.95  8.15  8.3  8.45  8.65  8.8  9  9.15  9.35  9.5  9.7  9.9  10.05  10.25  10.45  10.65  10.85  11.05

FOR EDGE LIFT   0.07 ,   OPTIC DIAMETERS   9.6  -  10.4 ,   ZONAL CURVATURES ARE
 7.75  7.9  8.05  8.2  8.4  8.55  8.75  8.9  9.05  9.25  9.4  9.6  9.8  9.95  10.15  10.35  10.55  10.7  10.9

FOR EDGE LIFT   0.07 ,   OPTIC DIAMETERS   9.8  -  10.6 ,   ZONAL CURVATURES ARE
 7.65  7.85  8  8.15  8.3  8.5  8.65  8.8  9  9.15  9.35  9.5  9.7  9.85  10.05  10.25  10.4  10.6  10.8

FOR EDGE LIFT   0.07 ,   OPTIC DIAMETERS   10.  -  10.8 ,   ZONAL CURVATURES ARE
 7.6  7.75  7.9  8.1  8.25  8.4  8.55  8.75  8.9  9.05  9.25  9.4  9.6  9.75  9.95  10.1  10.3  10.5  10.7

FOR EDGE LIFT   0.07 ,   OPTIC DIAMETERS   10.2  -  11. ,   ZONAL CURVATURES ARE
 7.55  7.7  7.85  8  8.15  8.35  8.5  8.65  8.8  9  9.15  9.35  9.5  9.65  9.85  10  10.2  10.4  10.55

FOR EDGE LIFT   0.07 ,   OPTIC DIAMETERS   10.4  -  11.2 ,   ZONAL CURVATURES ARE
 7.5  7.65  7.8  7.95  8.1  8.25  8.4  8.6  8.75  8.9  9.05  9.25  9.4  9.6  9.75  9.95  10.1  10.3  10.45
```

FOR EDGE LIFT 0.08 , OPTIC DIAMETERS 7 - 7.8 , ZONAL CURVATURES ARE

9.5 9.75 10 10.2 10.45 10.75 11 11.25 11.5 11.8 12.1 12.35 12.65 12.95 13.25 13.55 13.85 14.2 14.5

FOR EDGE LIFT 0.08 , OPTIC DIAMETERS 7.2 - 8 , ZONAL CURVATURES ARE

9.3 9.55 9.8 10 10.25 10.5 10.75 11 11.25 11.55 11.8 12.1 12.35 12.65 12.95 13.25 13.55 13.85 14.15

FOR EDGE LIFT 0.08 , OPTIC DIAMETERS 7.4 - 8.2 , ZONAL CURVATURES ARE

9.15 9.35 9.6 9.85 10.05 10.3 10.55 10.8 11.05 11.3 11.55 11.8 12.1 12.35 12.65 12.9 13.2 13.5 13.8

FOR EDGE LIFT 0.08 , OPTIC DIAMETERS 7.6 - 8.4 , ZONAL CURVATURES ARE

9 9.2 9.45 9.65 9.9 10.1 10.35 10.6 10.85 11.05 11.3 11.6 11.85 12.1 12.35 12.65 12.9 13.2 13.5

FOR EDGE LIFT 0.08 , OPTIC DIAMETERS 7.8 - 8.6 , ZONAL CURVATURES ARE

8.85 9.05 9.25 9.5 9.7 9.95 10.15 10.4 10.65 10.85 11.1 11.35 11.6 11.85 12.1 12.4 12.65 12.9 13.2

FOR EDGE LIFT 0.08 , OPTIC DIAMETERS 8. - 8.8 , ZONAL CURVATURES ARE

8.7 8.9 9.1 9.35 9.55 9.75 10 10.2 10.45 10.65 10.9 11.15 11.4 11.65 11.9 12.15 12.4 12.65 12.95

FOR EDGE LIFT 0.08 , OPTIC DIAMETERS 8.2 - 9. , ZONAL CURVATURES ARE

8.6 8.8 9 9.2 9.4 9.6 9.85 10.05 10.25 10.5 10.7 10.95 11.2 11.45 11.7 11.9 12.15 12.45 12.7

FOR EDGE LIFT 0.08 , OPTIC DIAMETERS 8.4 - 9.2 , ZONAL CURVATURES ARE

8.45 8.65 8.85 9.05 9.25 9.45 9.7 9.9 10.1 10.35 10.55 10.8 11 11.25 11.5 11.7 11.95 12.2 12.45

FOR EDGE LIFT 0.08 , OPTIC DIAMETERS 8.6 - 9.4 , ZONAL CURVATURES ARE

8.35 8.55 8.75 8.95 9.15 9.35 9.55 9.75 9.95 10.15 10.4 10.6 10.85 11.05 11.3 11.5 11.75 12 12.25

```
FOR EDGE LIFT   0.08 ,   OPTIC DIAMETERS   8.8  -  9.6 ,   ZONAL CURVATURES ARE
 8.25  8.45  8.6  8.8  9  9.2  9.4  9.6  9.8  10  10.25  10.45  10.65  10.9  11.1  11.35  11.55  11.8  12.05

FOR EDGE LIFT   0.08 ,   OPTIC DIAMETERS   9.  -  9.8 ,   ZONAL CURVATURES ARE
 8.15  8.35  8.5  8.7  8.9  9.1  9.3  9.5  9.7  9.9  10.1  10.3  10.5  10.75  10.95  11.15  11.4  11.6  11.85

FOR EDGE LIFT   0.08 ,   OPTIC DIAMETERS   9.2  -  10. ,   ZONAL CURVATURES ARE
 8.05  8.25  8.4  8.6  8.8  8.95  9.15  9.35  9.55  9.75  9.95  10.15  10.35  10.6  10.8  11  11.25  11.45  11.65

FOR EDGE LIFT   0.08 ,   OPTIC DIAMETERS   9.4  -  10.2 ,   ZONAL CURVATURES ARE
 7.95  8.15  8.3  8.5  8.7  8.85  9.05  9.25  9.45  9.65  9.85  10.05  10.25  10.45  10.65  10.85  11.05  11.3  11.5

FOR EDGE LIFT   0.08 ,   OPTIC DIAMETERS   9.6  -  10.4 ,   ZONAL CURVATURES ARE
 7.9  8.05  8.2  8.4  8.6  8.75  8.95  9.15  9.3  9.5  9.7  9.9  10.1  10.3  10.5  10.7  10.9  11.15  11.35

FOR EDGE LIFT   0.08 ,   OPTIC DIAMETERS   9.8  -  10.6 ,   ZONAL CURVATURES ARE
 7.8  7.95  8.15  8.3  8.5  8.65  8.85  9.05  9.2  9.4  9.6  9.8  10  10.2  10.4  10.6  10.8  11  11.2

FOR EDGE LIFT   0.08 ,   OPTIC DIAMETERS   10.  -  10.8 ,   ZONAL CURVATURES ARE
 7.7  7.9  8.05  8.25  8.4  8.55  8.75  8.95  9.1  9.3  9.5  9.65  9.85  10.05  10.25  10.45  10.65  10.85  11.05

FOR EDGE LIFT   0.08 ,   OPTIC DIAMETERS   10.2  -  11. ,   ZONAL CURVATURES ARE
 7.65  7.8  8  8.15  8.3  8.5  8.65  8.85  9  9.2  9.4  9.55  9.75  9.95  10.15  10.35  10.5  10.7  10.95

FOR EDGE LIFT   0.08 ,   OPTIC DIAMETERS   10.4  -  11.2 ,   ZONAL CURVATURES ARE
 7.6  7.75  7.9  8.05  8.25  8.4  8.6  8.75  8.9  9.1  9.3  9.45  9.65  9.85  10  10.2  10.4  10.6  10.8
```

```
FOR EDGE LIFT   0.09 ,   OPTIC DIAMETERS   7  -  7.8 ,    ZONAL CURVATURES ARE
 10  10.3  10.55  10.85  11.15  11.4  11.7  12.05  12.35  12.65  13  13.35  13.7  14.05  14.4  14.75  15.15  15.55  15.95

FOR EDGE LIFT   0.09 ,   OPTIC DIAMETERS   7.2  -  8 ,    ZONAL CURVATURES ARE
 9.8  10.05  10.3  10.6  10.85  11.15  11.45  11.7  12  12.35  12.65  12.95  13.3  13.65  14  14.35  14.7  15.05  15.45

FOR EDGE LIFT   0.09 ,   OPTIC DIAMETERS   7.4  -  8.2 ,    ZONAL CURVATURES ARE
 9.55  9.8  10.1  10.35  10.6  10.9  11.15  11.45  11.75  12  12.3  12.65  12.95  13.25  13.6  13.95  14.3  14.65  15

FOR EDGE LIFT   0.09 ,   OPTIC DIAMETERS   7.6  -  8.4 ,    ZONAL CURVATURES ARE
 9.35  9.6  9.85  10.1  10.35  10.65  10.9  11.2  11.45  11.75  12.05  12.3  12.65  12.95  13.25  13.55  13.9  14.25  14.55

FOR EDGE LIFT   0.09 ,   OPTIC DIAMETERS   7.8  -  8.6 ,    ZONAL CURVATURES ARE
 9.2  9.45  9.65  9.9  10.15  10.4  10.65  10.95  11.2  11.5  11.75  12.05  12.35  12.6  12.95  13.25  13.55  13.85  14.2

FOR EDGE LIFT   0.09 ,   OPTIC DIAMETERS   8.  -  8.8 ,    ZONAL CURVATURES ARE
 9.05  9.25  9.5  9.7  9.95  10.2  10.45  10.7  10.95  11.25  11.5  11.8  12.05  12.35  12.65  12.95  13.25  13.55  13.85

FOR EDGE LIFT   0.09 ,   OPTIC DIAMETERS   8.2  -  9. ,    ZONAL CURVATURES ARE
 8.85  9.1  9.3  9.55  9.8  10  10.25  10.5  10.75  11  11.25  11.55  11.8  12.1  12.35  12.65  12.95  13.25  13.55

FOR EDGE LIFT   0.09 ,   OPTIC DIAMETERS   8.4  -  9.2 ,    ZONAL CURVATURES ARE
 8.75  8.95  9.15  9.4  9.6  9.85  10.1  10.3  10.55  10.8  11.05  11.3  11.55  11.85  12.1  12.4  12.65  12.95  13.25

FOR EDGE LIFT   0.09 ,   OPTIC DIAMETERS   8.6  -  9.4 ,    ZONAL CURVATURES ARE
 8.6  8.8  9  9.25  9.45  9.65  9.9  10.15  10.35  10.6  10.85  11.1  11.35  11.6  11.85  12.15  12.4  12.7  12.95
```

FOR EDGE LIFT 0.09 , OPTIC DIAMETERS 8.8 - 9.6 , ZONAL CURVATURES ARE

8.45 8.65 8.85 9.1 9.3 9.5 9.75 9.95 10.2 10.45 10.65 10.9 11.15 11.4 11.65 11.9 12.15 12.45 12.7

FOR EDGE LIFT 0.09 , OPTIC DIAMETERS 9. - 9.8 , ZONAL CURVATURES ARE

8.35 8.55 8.75 8.95 9.15 9.35 9.6 9.8 10.05 10.25 10.5 10.7 10.95 11.2 11.45 11.7 11.95 12.2 12.45

FOR EDGE LIFT 0.09 , OPTIC DIAMETERS 9.2 - 10. , ZONAL CURVATURES ARE

8.25 8.4 8.6 8.8 9.05 9.25 9.45 9.65 9.9 10.1 10.3 10.55 10.8 11 11.25 11.5 11.75 12 12.25

FOR EDGE LIFT 0.09 , OPTIC DIAMETERS 9.4 - 10.2 , ZONAL CURVATURES ARE

8.1 8.3 8.5 8.7 8.9 9.1 9.3 9.5 9.75 9.95 10.15 10.4 10.6 10.85 11.05 11.3 11.55 11.8 12.05

FOR EDGE LIFT 0.09 , OPTIC DIAMETERS 9.6 - 10.4 , ZONAL CURVATURES ARE

8 8.2 8.4 8.6 8.8 9 9.2 9.4 9.6 9.8 10 10.25 10.45 10.7 10.9 11.15 11.35 11.6 11.85

FOR EDGE LIFT 0.09 , OPTIC DIAMETERS 9.8 - 10.6 , ZONAL CURVATURES ARE

7.95 8.1 8.3 8.5 8.65 8.85 9.05 9.25 9.45 9.65 9.9 10.1 10.3 10.5 10.75 10.95 11.2 11.4 11.65

FOR EDGE LIFT 0.09 , OPTIC DIAMETERS 10. - 10.8 , ZONAL CURVATURES ARE

7.85 8 8.2 8.4 8.55 8.75 8.95 9.15 9.35 9.55 9.75 9.95 10.15 10.35 10.6 10.8 11.05 11.25 11.5

FOR EDGE LIFT 0.09 , OPTIC DIAMETERS 10.2 - 11. , ZONAL CURVATURES ARE

7.75 7.95 8.1 8.3 8.45 8.65 8.85 9.05 9.25 9.4 9.6 9.8 10.05 10.25 10.45 10.65 10.9 11.1 11.3

FOR EDGE LIFT 0.09 , OPTIC DIAMETERS 10.4 - 11.2 , ZONAL CURVATURES ARE

7.7 7.85 8 8.2 8.4 8.55 8.75 8.95 9.1 9.3 9.5 9.7 9.9 10.1 10.3 10.5 10.75 10.95 11.15

```
FOR EDGE LIFT   0.1 ,   OPTIC DIAMETERS   7  -  7.8 ,    ZONAL CURVATURES ARE
 10.6  10.9  11.2  11.55  11.9  12.25  12.6  12.95  13.3  13.7  14.1  14.5  14.95  15.35  15.8  16.25  16.75  17.2  17.7

FOR EDGE LIFT   0.1 ,   OPTIC DIAMETERS   7.2  -  8 ,    ZONAL CURVATURES ARE
 10.3  10.6  10.9  11.2  11.55  11.85  12.2  12.55  12.9  13.25  13.65  14.05  14.4  14.8  15.25  15.65  16.1  16.55  17.05

FOR EDGE LIFT   0.1 ,   OPTIC DIAMETERS   7.4  -  8.2 ,    ZONAL CURVATURES ARE
 10.05  10.35  10.6  10.9  11.25  11.55  11.85  12.2  12.55  12.85  13.25  13.6  13.95  14.35  14.75  15.15  15.55  16  16.4

FOR EDGE LIFT   0.1 ,   OPTIC DIAMETERS   7.6  -  8.4 ,    ZONAL CURVATURES ARE
 9.8  10.1  10.35  10.65  10.95  11.25  11.55  11.85  12.2  12.5  12.85  13.2  13.55  13.9  14.3  14.65  15.05  15.45  15.85

FOR EDGE LIFT   0.1 ,   OPTIC DIAMETERS   7.8  -  8.6 ,    ZONAL CURVATURES ARE
 9.6  9.85  10.1  10.4  10.7  10.95  11.25  11.55  11.85  12.2  12.5  12.85  13.15  13.5  13.85  14.25  14.6  15  15.35

FOR EDGE LIFT   0.1 ,   OPTIC DIAMETERS   8.  -  8.8 ,    ZONAL CURVATURES ARE
 9.4  9.65  9.9  10.15  10.45  10.7  11  11.3  11.6  11.9  12.2  12.5  12.8  13.15  13.5  13.85  14.2  14.55  14.9

FOR EDGE LIFT   0.1 ,   OPTIC DIAMETERS   8.2  -  9. ,    ZONAL CURVATURES ARE
 9.2  9.45  9.7  9.95  10.2  10.45  10.75  11  11.3  11.6  11.9  12.2  12.5  12.8  13.15  13.5  13.8  14.15  14.5

FOR EDGE LIFT   0.1 ,   OPTIC DIAMETERS   8.4  -  9.2 ,    ZONAL CURVATURES ARE
 9  9.25  9.5  9.75  10  10.25  10.5  10.8  11.05  11.35  11.65  11.9  12.2  12.5  12.85  13.15  13.45  13.8  14.15

FOR EDGE LIFT   0.1 ,   OPTIC DIAMETERS   8.6  -  9.4 ,    ZONAL CURVATURES ARE
 8.85  9.1  9.3  9.55  9.8  10.05  10.3  10.55  10.85  11.1  11.4  11.65  11.95  12.25  12.55  12.85  13.15  13.45  13.8
```

```
FOR EDGE LIFT   0.1 ,   OPTIC DIAMETERS   8.8  -  9.6 ,    ZONAL CURVATURES ARE
 8.7  8.95  9.15  9.4  9.6  9.85  10.1  10.35  10.6  10.9  11.15  11.4  11.7  11.95  12.25  12.55  12.85  13.15  13.45

FOR EDGE LIFT   0.1 ,   OPTIC DIAMETERS   9.  -  9.8 ,    ZONAL CURVATURES ARE
 8.55  8.8  9  9.2  9.45  9.7  9.95  10.15  10.4  10.65  10.95  11.2  11.45  11.75  12  12.3  12.6  12.85  13.15

FOR EDGE LIFT   0.1 ,   OPTIC DIAMETERS   9.2  -  10. ,    ZONAL CURVATURES ARE
 8.45  8.65  8.85  9.05  9.3  9.5  9.75  10  10.25  10.5  10.75  11  11.25  11.5  11.75  12.05  12.3  12.6  12.9

FOR EDGE LIFT   0.1 ,   OPTIC DIAMETERS   9.4  -  10.2 ,    ZONAL CURVATURES ARE
 8.3  8.5  8.7  8.95  9.15  9.35  9.6  9.8  10.05  10.3  10.55  10.8  11.05  11.3  11.55  11.8  12.1  12.35  12.65

FOR EDGE LIFT   0.1 ,   OPTIC DIAMETERS   9.6  -  10.4 ,    ZONAL CURVATURES ARE
 8.2  8.4  8.6  8.8  9  9.2  9.45  9.65  9.9  10.1  10.35  10.6  10.85  11.1  11.35  11.6  11.85  12.15  12.4

FOR EDGE LIFT   0.1 ,   OPTIC DIAMETERS   9.8  -  10.6 ,    ZONAL CURVATURES ARE
 8.05  8.25  8.45  8.65  8.9  9.1  9.3  9.5  9.75  9.95  10.2  10.4  10.65  10.9  11.15  11.4  11.65  11.9  12.15

FOR EDGE LIFT   0.1 ,   OPTIC DIAMETERS   10.  -  10.8 ,    ZONAL CURVATURES ARE
 7.95  8.15  8.35  8.55  8.75  8.95  9.15  9.4  9.6  9.8  10.05  10.25  10.5  10.75  10.95  11.2  11.45  11.7  11.95

FOR EDGE LIFT   0.1 ,   OPTIC DIAMETERS   10.2  -  11. ,    ZONAL CURVATURES ARE
 7.85  8.05  8.25  8.45  8.65  8.85  9.05  9.25  9.45  9.65  9.9  10.1  10.35  10.55  10.8  11.05  11.25  11.5  11.75

FOR EDGE LIFT   0.1 ,   OPTIC DIAMETERS   10.4  -  11.2 ,    ZONAL CURVATURES ARE
 7.8  7.95  8.15  8.35  8.55  8.7  8.9  9.1  9.35  9.55  9.75  9.95  10.2  10.4  10.65  10.85  11.1  11.35  11.55
```

```
FOR EDGE LIFT   0.11 ,   OPTIC DIAMETERS   7 - 7.8 ,    ZONAL CURVATURES ARE
 11.25  11.6  12  12.4  12.75  13.2  13.6  14.05  14.5  14.95  15.45  15.95  16.45  17  17.55  18.1  18.7  19.3  19.95

FOR EDGE LIFT   0.11 ,   OPTIC DIAMETERS   7.2 - 8 ,    ZONAL CURVATURES ARE
 10.9  11.25  11.6  11.95  12.35  12.7  13.1  13.55  13.95  14.4  14.85  15.3  15.8  16.25  16.8  17.3  17.85  18.45  19

FOR EDGE LIFT   0.11 ,   OPTIC DIAMETERS   7.4 - 8.2 ,    ZONAL CURVATURES ARE
 10.6  10.9  11.25  11.6  11.95  12.3  12.7  13.05  13.45  13.85  14.3  14.75  15.2  15.65  16.1  16.6  17.1  17.65  18.2

FOR EDGE LIFT   0.11 ,   OPTIC DIAMETERS   7.6 - 8.4 ,    ZONAL CURVATURES ARE
 10.3  10.6  10.9  11.25  11.6  11.95  12.3  12.65  13.05  13.4  13.8  14.2  14.65  15.05  15.5  16  16.45  16.95  17.45

FOR EDGE LIFT   0.11 ,   OPTIC DIAMETERS   7.8 - 8.6 ,    ZONAL CURVATURES ARE
 10  10.3  10.65  10.95  11.25  11.6  11.95  12.25  12.65  13  13.35  13.75  14.15  14.55  15  15.4  15.85  16.3  16.8

FOR EDGE LIFT   0.11 ,   OPTIC DIAMETERS   8. - 8.8 ,    ZONAL CURVATURES ARE
 9.8  10.05  10.35  10.65  10.95  11.3  11.6  11.95  12.25  12.6  12.95  13.35  13.7  14.1  14.5  14.9  15.35  15.75  16.2

FOR EDGE LIFT   0.11 ,   OPTIC DIAMETERS   8.2 - 9. ,    ZONAL CURVATURES ARE
 9.55  9.85  10.1  10.4  10.7  11  11.3  11.6  11.95  12.25  12.6  12.95  13.3  13.7  14.05  14.45  14.85  15.25  15.65

FOR EDGE LIFT   0.11 ,   OPTIC DIAMETERS   8.4 - 9.2 ,    ZONAL CURVATURES ARE
 9.35  9.6  9.9  10.15  10.45  10.7  11  11.3  11.65  11.95  12.3  12.6  12.95  13.3  13.65  14.05  14.4  14.8  15.2

FOR EDGE LIFT   0.11 ,   OPTIC DIAMETERS   8.6 - 9.4 ,    ZONAL CURVATURES ARE
 9.15  9.4  9.65  9.95  10.2  10.5  10.75  11.05  11.35  11.65  11.95  12.3  12.6  12.95  13.3  13.65  14  14.35  14.75
```

FOR EDGE LIFT 0.11 , OPTIC DIAMETERS 8.8 - 9.6 , ZONAL CURVATURES ARE

8.95 9.2 9.45 9.7 10 10.25 10.55 10.8 11.1 11.4 11.7 12 12.3 12.65 12.95 13.3 13.65 14 14.35

FOR EDGE LIFT 0.11 , OPTIC DIAMETERS 9. - 9.8 , ZONAL CURVATURES ARE

8.8 9.05 9.3 9.55 9.8 10.05 10.3 10.6 10.85 11.15 11.4 11.7 12 12.35 12.65 12.95 13.3 13.65 14

FOR EDGE LIFT 0.11 , OPTIC DIAMETERS 9.2 - 10. , ZONAL CURVATURES ARE

8.65 8.85 9.1 9.35 9.6 9.85 10.1 10.35 10.65 10.9 11.2 11.45 11.75 12.05 12.35 12.65 13 13.3 13.65

FOR EDGE LIFT 0.11 , OPTIC DIAMETERS 9.4 - 10.2 , ZONAL CURVATURES ARE

8.5 8.7 8.95 9.2 9.4 9.65 9.9 10.15 10.4 10.7 10.95 11.25 11.5 11.8 12.1 12.4 12.7 13 13.3

FOR EDGE LIFT 0.11 , OPTIC DIAMETERS 9.6 - 10.4 , ZONAL CURVATURES ARE

8.35 8.55 8.8 9 9.25 9.5 9.75 9.95 10.2 10.5 10.75 11 11.25 11.55 11.85 12.1 12.4 12.7 13

FOR EDGE LIFT 0.11 , OPTIC DIAMETERS 9.8 - 10.6 , ZONAL CURVATURES ARE

8.25 8.45 8.65 8.85 9.1 9.35 9.55 9.8 10.05 10.3 10.55 10.8 11.05 11.35 11.6 11.9 12.15 12.45 12.75

FOR EDGE LIFT 0.11 , OPTIC DIAMETERS 10. - 10.8 , ZONAL CURVATURES ARE

8.1 8.3 8.5 8.75 8.95 9.15 9.4 9.65 9.85 10.1 10.35 10.6 10.85 11.1 11.4 11.65 11.95 12.2 12.5

FOR EDGE LIFT 0.11 , OPTIC DIAMETERS 10.2 - 11. , ZONAL CURVATURES ARE

8 8.2 8.4 8.6 8.8 9.05 9.25 9.5 9.7 9.95 10.2 10.4 10.65 10.9 11.15 11.45 11.7 11.95 12.25

FOR EDGE LIFT 0.11 , OPTIC DIAMETERS 10.4 - 11.2 , ZONAL CURVATURES ARE

7.9 8.1 8.3 8.5 8.7 8.9 9.1 9.35 9.55 9.8 10 10.25 10.5 10.75 11 11.25 11.5 11.75 12.05

```
FOR EDGE LIFT   0.12 ,   OPTIC DIAMETERS   7  -  7.8 ,   ZONAL CURVATURES ARE
 12.05  12.45  12.9  13.35  13.85  14.3  14.85  15.35  15.9  16.5  17.1  17.7  18.35  19.05  19.75  20.5  21.25  22.05  22.9

FOR EDGE LIFT   0.12 ,   OPTIC DIAMETERS   7.2  -  8 ,   ZONAL CURVATURES ARE
 11.6  12  12.4  12.85  13.25  13.75  14.2  14.7  15.2  15.75  16.3  16.85  17.45  18.05  18.7  19.4  20.1  20.8  21.55

FOR EDGE LIFT   0.12 ,   OPTIC DIAMETERS   7.4  -  8.2 ,   ZONAL CURVATURES ARE
 11.2  11.6  11.95  12.35  12.8  13.2  13.65  14.1  14.6  15.05  15.6  16.1  16.65  17.2  17.8  18.4  19.05  19.75  20.4

FOR EDGE LIFT   0.12 ,   OPTIC DIAMETERS   7.6  -  8.4 ,   ZONAL CURVATURES ARE
 10.85  11.2  11.55  11.95  12.35  12.75  13.15  13.6  14  14.5  14.95  15.45  15.95  16.5  17  17.6  18.15  18.8  19.4

FOR EDGE LIFT   0.12 ,   OPTIC DIAMETERS   7.8  -  8.6 ,   ZONAL CURVATURES ARE
 10.5  10.85  11.2  11.55  11.95  12.3  12.7  13.1  13.5  13.95  14.4  14.85  15.35  15.8  16.3  16.85  17.4  17.95  18.55

FOR EDGE LIFT   0.12 ,   OPTIC DIAMETERS   8.  -  8.8 ,   ZONAL CURVATURES ARE
 10.2  10.55  10.85  11.2  11.55  11.9  12.3  12.7  13.05  13.45  13.9  14.3  14.75  15.25  15.7  16.2  16.7  17.2  17.75

FOR EDGE LIFT   0.12 ,   OPTIC DIAMETERS   8.2  -  9. ,   ZONAL CURVATURES ARE
 9.95  10.25  10.55  10.9  11.25  11.55  11.9  12.3  12.65  13.05  13.45  13.85  14.25  14.7  15.15  15.6  16.1  16.55  17.05

FOR EDGE LIFT   0.12 ,   OPTIC DIAMETERS   8.4  -  9.2 ,   ZONAL CURVATURES ARE
 9.7  10  10.3  10.6  10.9  11.25  11.6  11.95  12.3  12.65  13  13.4  13.8  14.2  14.65  15.05  15.5  16  16.45

FOR EDGE LIFT   0.12 ,   OPTIC DIAMETERS   8.6  -  9.4 ,   ZONAL CURVATURES ARE
 9.45  9.75  10.05  10.35  10.65  10.95  11.3  11.6  11.95  12.3  12.65  13  13.4  13.8  14.2  14.6  15  15.45  15.9
```

```
FOR EDGE LIFT   0.12 ,   OPTIC DIAMETERS   8.8  -  9.6 ,    ZONAL CURVATURES ARE
 9.25  9.55  9.8  10.1  10.4  10.7  11  11.3  11.65  11.95  12.3  12.65  13  13.4  13.75  14.15  14.55  14.95  15.4

FOR EDGE LIFT   0.12 ,   OPTIC DIAMETERS   9.  -  9.8 ,    ZONAL CURVATURES ARE
 9.05  9.3  9.6  9.85  10.15  10.45  10.75  11.05  11.35  11.65  12  12.3  12.65  13  13.35  13.75  14.1  14.5  14.9

FOR EDGE LIFT   0.12 ,   OPTIC DIAMETERS   9.2  -  10. ,    ZONAL CURVATURES ARE
 8.85  9.15  9.4  9.65  9.9  10.2  10.5  10.75  11.05  11.35  11.7  12  12.35  12.65  13  13.35  13.75  14.1  14.5

FOR EDGE LIFT   0.12 ,   OPTIC DIAMETERS   9.4  -  10.2 ,    ZONAL CURVATURES ARE
 8.7  8.95  9.2  9.45  9.7  10  10.25  10.55  10.8  11.1  11.4  11.7  12.05  12.35  12.7  13.05  13.4  13.75  14.1

FOR EDGE LIFT   0.12 ,   OPTIC DIAMETERS   9.6  -  10.4 ,    ZONAL CURVATURES ARE
 8.55  8.8  9  9.25  9.5  9.8  10.05  10.3  10.6  10.85  11.15  11.45  11.75  12.05  12.4  12.7  13.05  13.4  13.75

FOR EDGE LIFT   0.12 ,   OPTIC DIAMETERS   9.8  -  10.6 ,    ZONAL CURVATURES ARE
 8.4  8.6  8.85  9.1  9.35  9.6  9.85  10.1  10.35  10.65  10.9  11.2  11.5  11.8  12.1  12.4  12.75  13.05  13.4

FOR EDGE LIFT   0.12 ,   OPTIC DIAMETERS   10.  -  10.8 ,    ZONAL CURVATURES ARE
 8.25  8.45  8.7  8.95  9.15  9.4  9.65  9.9  10.15  10.45  10.7  11  11.25  11.55  11.85  12.15  12.45  12.75  13.1

FOR EDGE LIFT   0.12 ,   OPTIC DIAMETERS   10.2  -  11. ,    ZONAL CURVATURES ARE
 8.1  8.35  8.55  8.8  9  9.25  9.5  9.75  10  10.25  10.5  10.75  11.05  11.3  11.6  11.9  12.2  12.5  12.8

FOR EDGE LIFT   0.12 ,   OPTIC DIAMETERS   10.4  -  11.2 ,    ZONAL CURVATURES ARE
 8  8.2  8.4  8.65  8.85  9.1  9.3  9.55  9.8  10.05  10.3  10.55  10.8  11.1  11.35  11.65  11.95  12.25  12.55
```

```
FOR EDGE LIFT   0.13 ,   OPTIC DIAMETERS   7  -  7.8 ,    ZONAL CURVATURES ARE
 12.95  13.45  14  14.55  15.1  15.7  16.35  17  17.65  18.4  19.15  19.95  20.8  21.7  22.6  23.6  24.65  25.75  26.95

FOR EDGE LIFT   0.13 ,   OPTIC DIAMETERS   7.2  -  8 ,    ZONAL CURVATURES ARE
 12.4  12.85  13.35  13.85  14.4  14.95  15.5  16.1  16.75  17.4  18.05  18.8  19.55  20.35  21.15  22.05  22.95  23.95  25

FOR EDGE LIFT   0.13 ,   OPTIC DIAMETERS   7.4  -  8.2 ,    ZONAL CURVATURES ARE
 11.9  12.35  12.8  13.25  13.75  14.25  14.8  15.35  15.9  16.5  17.15  17.8  18.5  19.2  19.95  20.7  21.55  22.4  23.35

FOR EDGE LIFT   0.13 ,   OPTIC DIAMETERS   7.6  -  8.4 ,    ZONAL CURVATURES ARE
 11.5  11.9  12.3  12.75  13.2  13.65  14.15  14.65  15.2  15.75  16.35  16.95  17.55  18.2  18.9  19.6  20.35  21.1  21.95

FOR EDGE LIFT   0.13 ,   OPTIC DIAMETERS   7.8  -  8.6 ,    ZONAL CURVATURES ARE
 11.1  11.45  11.85  12.3  12.7  13.15  13.6  14.1  14.55  15.1  15.6  16.15  16.75  17.35  17.95  18.6  19.3  20  20.75

FOR EDGE LIFT   0.13 ,   OPTIC DIAMETERS   8.  -  8.8 ,    ZONAL CURVATURES ARE
 10.7  11.1  11.45  11.85  12.25  12.65  13.1  13.55  14  14.5  15  15.5  16  16.55  17.15  17.75  18.35  19  19.7

FOR EDGE LIFT   0.13 ,   OPTIC DIAMETERS   8.2  -  9. ,    ZONAL CURVATURES ARE
 10.4  10.75  11.1  11.45  11.85  12.25  12.65  13.05  13.5  13.95  14.4  14.9  15.4  15.9  16.45  17  17.55  18.15  18.75

FOR EDGE LIFT   0.13 ,   OPTIC DIAMETERS   8.4  -  9.2 ,    ZONAL CURVATURES ARE
 10.1  10.45  10.75  11.1  11.5  11.85  12.25  12.65  13.05  13.45  13.9  14.35  14.8  15.3  15.8  16.3  16.85  17.4  17.95

FOR EDGE LIFT   0.13 ,   OPTIC DIAMETERS   8.6  -  9.4 ,    ZONAL CURVATURES ARE
 9.85  10.15  10.45  10.8  11.15  11.5  11.85  12.25  12.6  13  13.45  13.85  14.3  14.75  15.2  15.7  16.2  16.7  17.25
```

```
FOR EDGE LIFT   0.13 ,   OPTIC DIAMETERS   8.8  -  9.6 ,    ZONAL CURVATURES ARE
 9.6  9.9  10.2  10.5  10.85  11.15  11.5  11.85  12.25  12.6  13  13.4  13.8  14.25  14.7  15.15  15.6  16.1  16.6

FOR EDGE LIFT   0.13 ,   OPTIC DIAMETERS   9.  -  9.8 ,    ZONAL CURVATURES ARE
 9.35  9.65  9.95  10.25  10.55  10.85  11.2  11.55  11.9  12.25  12.6  13  13.4  13.8  14.2  14.65  15.1  15.55  16

FOR EDGE LIFT   0.13 ,   OPTIC DIAMETERS   9.2  -  10. ,    ZONAL CURVATURES ARE
 9.15  9.4  9.7  10  10.3  10.6  10.9  11.25  11.55  11.9  12.25  12.6  13  13.4  13.8  14.2  14.6  15.05  15.5

FOR EDGE LIFT   0.13 ,   OPTIC DIAMETERS   9.4  -  10.2 ,    ZONAL CURVATURES ARE
 8.95  9.2  9.45  9.75  10.05  10.35  10.65  10.95  11.25  11.6  11.95  12.3  12.65  13  13.4  13.75  14.15  14.6  15

FOR EDGE LIFT   0.13 ,   OPTIC DIAMETERS   9.6  -  10.4 ,    ZONAL CURVATURES ARE
 8.75  9  9.25  9.55  9.8  10.1  10.4  10.7  11  11.3  11.65  11.95  12.3  12.65  13  13.4  13.75  14.15  14.55

FOR EDGE LIFT   0.13 ,   OPTIC DIAMETERS   9.8  -  10.6 ,    ZONAL CURVATURES ARE
 8.55  8.8  9.05  9.35  9.6  9.85  10.15  10.45  10.75  11.05  11.35  11.65  12  12.35  12.65  13.05  13.4  13.75  14.15

FOR EDGE LIFT   0.13 ,   OPTIC DIAMETERS   10.  -  10.8 ,    ZONAL CURVATURES ARE
 8.4  8.65  8.9  9.15  9.4  9.65  9.95  10.2  10.5  10.8  11.1  11.4  11.7  12.05  12.35  12.7  13.05  13.4  13.75

FOR EDGE LIFT   0.13 ,   OPTIC DIAMETERS   10.2  -  11. ,    ZONAL CURVATURES ARE
 8.25  8.5  8.75  8.95  9.2  9.45  9.75  10  10.3  10.55  10.85  11.15  11.45  11.75  12.05  12.4  12.75  13.05  13.4

FOR EDGE LIFT   0.13 ,   OPTIC DIAMETERS   10.4  -  11.2 ,    ZONAL CURVATURES ARE
 8.1  8.35  8.6  8.8  9.05  9.3  9.55  9.8  10.05  10.35  10.6  10.9  11.2  11.5  11.8  12.1  12.45  12.75  13.1
```

```
FOR EDGE LIFT    0.14 ,    OPTIC DIAMETERS    7  -  7.8 ,     ZONAL CURVATURES ARE
 14.05  14.65  15.3  15.95  16.65  17.4  18.2  19.05  19.9  20.85  21.85  22.9  24.05  25.25  26.55  27.9  29.4  31.05  32.8

FOR EDGE LIFT    0.14 ,    OPTIC DIAMETERS    7.2  -  8 ,     ZONAL CURVATURES ARE
 13.35  13.9  14.5  15.1  15.75  16.4  17.1  17.85  18.65  19.5  20.35  21.3  22.25  23.3  24.45  25.6  26.9  28.25  29.7

FOR EDGE LIFT    0.14 ,    OPTIC DIAMETERS    7.4  -  8.2 ,     ZONAL CURVATURES ARE
 12.75  13.25  13.8  14.35  14.95  15.55  16.2  16.85  17.55  18.3  19.1  19.9  20.8  21.7  22.7  23.75  24.85  26  27.25

FOR EDGE LIFT    0.14 ,    OPTIC DIAMETERS    7.6  -  8.4 ,     ZONAL CURVATURES ARE
 12.2  12.7  13.15  13.7  14.25  14.8  15.4  16  16.65  17.3  18  18.75  19.55  20.35  21.25  22.15  23.1  24.15  25.25

FOR EDGE LIFT    0.14 ,    OPTIC DIAMETERS    7.8  -  8.6 ,     ZONAL CURVATURES ARE
 11.7  12.15  12.65  13.1  13.6  14.15  14.65  15.25  15.8  16.45  17.1  17.75  18.45  19.2  20  20.8  21.7  22.6  23.55

FOR EDGE LIFT    0.14 ,    OPTIC DIAMETERS    8.  -  8.8 ,     ZONAL CURVATURES ARE
 11.3  11.7  12.15  12.6  13.05  13.55  14.05  14.55  15.1  15.7  16.25  16.9  17.55  18.2  18.9  19.65  20.45  21.25  22.1

FOR EDGE LIFT    0.14 ,    OPTIC DIAMETERS    8.2  -  9. ,     ZONAL CURVATURES ARE
 10.9  11.3  11.7  12.1  12.55  13  13.5  13.95  14.45  15  15.55  16.1  16.7  17.35  18  18.65  19.35  20.1  20.9

FOR EDGE LIFT    0.14 ,    OPTIC DIAMETERS    8.4  -  9.2 ,     ZONAL CURVATURES ARE
 10.55  10.9  11.3  11.7  12.1  12.55  12.95  13.45  13.9  14.4  14.9  15.45  16  16.55  17.15  17.8  18.45  19.1  19.85

FOR EDGE LIFT    0.14 ,    OPTIC DIAMETERS    8.6  -  9.4 ,     ZONAL CURVATURES ARE
 10.25  10.6  10.95  11.3  11.7  12.1  12.5  12.95  13.4  13.85  14.35  14.85  15.35  15.9  16.45  17  17.6  18.25  18.9
```

```
FOR EDGE LIFT   0.14 ,   OPTIC DIAMETERS   8.8  -  9.6 ,    ZONAL CURVATURES ARE
 9.95  10.25  10.6  10.95  11.35  11.7  12.1  12.5  12.95  13.35  13.8  14.3  14.75  15.25  15.8  16.3  16.85  17.45  18.05

FOR EDGE LIFT   0.14 ,   OPTIC DIAMETERS   9.  -  9.8 ,    ZONAL CURVATURES ARE
 9.65  10  10.3  10.65  11  11.35  11.7  12.1  12.5  12.9  13.35  13.8  14.25  14.7  15.2  15.7  16.2  16.75  17.3

FOR EDGE LIFT   0.14 ,   OPTIC DIAMETERS   9.2  -  10. ,    ZONAL CURVATURES ARE
 9.4  9.7  10.05  10.35  10.7  11  11.4  11.75  12.1  12.5  12.9  13.3  13.75  14.2  14.65  15.15  15.6  16.1  16.65

FOR EDGE LIFT   0.14 ,   OPTIC DIAMETERS   9.4  -  10.2 ,    ZONAL CURVATURES ARE
 9.2  9.45  9.75  10.1  10.4  10.7  11.05  11.4  11.75  12.15  12.5  12.9  13.3  13.75  14.15  14.6  15.1  15.55  16.05

FOR EDGE LIFT   0.14 ,   OPTIC DIAMETERS   9.6  -  10.4 ,    ZONAL CURVATURES ARE
 8.95  9.25  9.55  9.85  10.15  10.45  10.75  11.1  11.45  11.8  12.15  12.55  12.9  13.3  13.7  14.15  14.6  15.05  15.5

FOR EDGE LIFT   0.14 ,   OPTIC DIAMETERS   9.8  -  10.6 ,    ZONAL CURVATURES ARE
 8.75  9.05  9.3  9.6  9.9  10.2  10.5  10.8  11.15  11.5  11.8  12.2  12.55  12.95  13.3  13.7  14.15  14.55  15

FOR EDGE LIFT   0.14 ,   OPTIC DIAMETERS   10.  -  10.8 ,    ZONAL CURVATURES ARE
 8.6  8.85  9.1  9.4  9.65  9.95  10.25  10.55  10.85  11.2  11.5  11.85  12.2  12.55  12.95  13.35  13.7  14.15  14.55

FOR EDGE LIFT   0.14 ,   OPTIC DIAMETERS   10.2  -  11. ,    ZONAL CURVATURES ARE
 8.4  8.65  8.9  9.2  9.45  9.75  10  10.3  10.6  10.9  11.25  11.55  11.9  12.25  12.6  12.95  13.35  13.7  14.1

FOR EDGE LIFT   0.14 ,   OPTIC DIAMETERS   10.4  -  11.2 ,    ZONAL CURVATURES ARE
 8.25  8.5  8.75  9  9.25  9.5  9.8  10.1  10.35  10.65  10.95  11.3  11.6  11.95  12.3  12.65  13  13.35  13.75
```

```
FOR EDGE LIFT   0.15 ,   OPTIC DIAMETERS   7  -  7.8 ,    ZONAL CURVATURES ARE
 15.35  16.1  16.9  17.75  18.6  19.55  20.6  21.7  22.85  24.1  25.45  26.9  28.5  30.25  32.15  34.25  36.55  39.1  41.95

FOR EDGE LIFT   0.15 ,   OPTIC DIAMETERS   7.2  -  8 ,    ZONAL CURVATURES ARE
 14.5  15.15  15.85  16.6  17.4  18.25  19.15  20.1  21.1  22.15  23.35  24.6  25.9  27.35  28.95  30.65  32.5  34.5  36.75

FOR EDGE LIFT   0.15 ,   OPTIC DIAMETERS   7.4  -  8.2 ,    ZONAL CURVATURES ARE
 13.7  14.35  14.95  15.65  16.35  17.1  17.9  18.75  19.65  20.6  21.6  22.65  23.8  25.05  26.4  27.8  29.35  31.05  32.85

FOR EDGE LIFT   0.15 ,   OPTIC DIAMETERS   7.6  -  8.4 ,    ZONAL CURVATURES ARE
 13.05  13.6  14.2  14.8  15.45  16.15  16.85  17.6  18.4  19.25  20.15  21.1  22.1  23.15  24.3  25.55  26.85  28.25  29.8

FOR EDGE LIFT   0.15 ,   OPTIC DIAMETERS   7.8  -  8.6 ,    ZONAL CURVATURES ARE
 12.45  13  13.5  14.1  14.65  15.3  15.95  16.65  17.35  18.1  18.9  19.75  20.65  21.6  22.6  23.65  24.8  26  27.3

FOR EDGE LIFT   0.15 ,   OPTIC DIAMETERS   8.  -  8.8 ,    ZONAL CURVATURES ARE
 11.95  12.4  12.9  13.45  14  14.55  15.15  15.8  16.45  17.1  17.85  18.6  19.4  20.25  21.15  22.1  23.1  24.15  25.3

FOR EDGE LIFT   0.15 ,   OPTIC DIAMETERS   8.2  -  9. ,    ZONAL CURVATURES ARE
 11.45  11.9  12.4  12.85  13.35  13.9  14.45  15.05  15.65  16.25  16.9  17.6  18.35  19.1  19.9  20.75  21.65  22.6  23.6

FOR EDGE LIFT   0.15 ,   OPTIC DIAMETERS   8.4  -  9.2 ,    ZONAL CURVATURES ARE
 11.05  11.45  11.9  12.35  12.85  13.3  13.85  14.35  14.9  15.5  16.1  16.75  17.4  18.1  18.85  19.6  20.4  21.25  22.15

FOR EDGE LIFT   0.15 ,   OPTIC DIAMETERS   8.6  -  9.4 ,    ZONAL CURVATURES ARE
 10.65  11.05  11.45  11.9  12.35  12.8  13.3  13.75  14.3  14.85  15.4  16  16.6  17.25  17.9  18.6  19.35  20.1  20.9
```

FOR EDGE LIFT 0.15 , OPTIC DIAMETERS 8.8 - 9.6 , ZONAL CURVATURES ARE

10.3 10.7 11.1 11.5 11.9 12.35 12.8 13.25 13.7 14.25 14.75 15.3 15.85 16.45 17.05 17.7 18.4 19.1 19.85

FOR EDGE LIFT 0.15 , OPTIC DIAMETERS 9. - 9.8 , ZONAL CURVATURES ARE

10 10.35 10.7 11.1 11.5 11.9 12.3 12.75 13.2 13.7 14.15 14.7 15.2 15.75 16.35 16.95 17.55 18.2 18.9

FOR EDGE LIFT 0.15 , OPTIC DIAMETERS 9.2 - 10. , ZONAL CURVATURES ARE

9.7 10.05 10.4 10.75 11.15 11.5 11.9 12.3 12.75 13.2 13.65 14.15 14.65 15.15 15.65 16.25 16.8 17.4 18.05

FOR EDGE LIFT 0.15 , OPTIC DIAMETERS 9.4 - 10.2 , ZONAL CURVATURES ARE

9.45 9.75 10.1 10.45 10.8 11.15 11.55 11.95 12.35 12.75 13.2 13.65 14.1 14.6 15.1 15.6 16.15 16.7 17.3

FOR EDGE LIFT 0.15 , OPTIC DIAMETERS 9.6 - 10.4 , ZONAL CURVATURES ARE

9.2 9.5 9.8 10.15 10.5 10.85 11.2 11.55 11.95 12.35 12.75 13.2 13.6 14.05 14.55 15.05 15.55 16.05 16.6

FOR EDGE LIFT 0.15 , OPTIC DIAMETERS 9.8 - 10.6 , ZONAL CURVATURES ARE

9 9.25 9.55 9.9 10.2 10.55 10.85 11.25 11.6 11.95 12.35 12.75 13.2 13.6 14.05 14.5 15 15.5 16

FOR EDGE LIFT 0.15 , OPTIC DIAMETERS 10. - 10.8 , ZONAL CURVATURES ARE

8.75 9.05 9.35 9.65 9.95 10.25 10.6 10.9 11.25 11.65 12 12.4 12.75 13.2 13.6 14.05 14.5 14.95 15.45

FOR EDGE LIFT 0.15 , OPTIC DIAMETERS 10.2 - 11. , ZONAL CURVATURES ARE

8.6 8.85 9.1 9.4 9.7 10 10.3 10.65 10.95 11.3 11.65 12.05 12.4 12.8 13.2 13.6 14.05 14.45 14.9

FOR EDGE LIFT 0.15 , OPTIC DIAMETERS 10.4 - 11.2 , ZONAL CURVATURES ARE

8.4 8.65 8.9 9.2 9.45 9.75 10.05 10.35 10.7 11 11.35 11.7 12.05 12.45 12.8 13.2 13.6 14.05 14.45

TABLE VII Back Peripheral Optic Radii (Zonal Curvatures) for the following:
BCOR 7.0 to 8.8 in 0.1 steps
Zone Width 0.5 Zone Inner Diameters 6.0 to 11.0 in 0.5 steps
Axial Edge Lift Components 0.01 to 0.15 in 0.01 steps

```
FOR EDGE LIFT   0.01 ,   OPTIC DIAMETERS   6 - 7 ,   ZONAL CURVATURES ARE
 7.2  7.35  7.45  7.55  7.65  7.75  7.85  8  8.1  8.2  8.3  8.45  8.55  8.65  8.75  8.85  9  9.1  9.2

FOR EDGE LIFT   0.01 ,   OPTIC DIAMETERS   6.5 - 7.5 ,   ZONAL CURVATURES ARE
 7.2  7.3  7.4  7.5  7.6  7.75  7.85  7.95  8.05  8.15  8.3  8.4  8.5  8.6  8.7  8.85  8.95  9.05  9.15

FOR EDGE LIFT   0.01 ,   OPTIC DIAMETERS   7 - 8 ,   ZONAL CURVATURES ARE
 7.15  7.25  7.4  7.5  7.6  7.7  7.8  7.9  8.05  8.15  8.25  8.35  8.45  8.55  8.7  8.8  8.9  9  9.1

FOR EDGE LIFT   0.01 ,   OPTIC DIAMETERS   7.5 - 8.5 ,   ZONAL CURVATURES ARE
 7.15  7.25  7.35  7.45  7.55  7.7  7.8  7.9  8  8.1  8.2  8.3  8.45  8.55  8.65  8.75  8.85  9  9.1

FOR EDGE LIFT   0.01 ,   OPTIC DIAMETERS   8 - 9 ,   ZONAL CURVATURES ARE
 7.1  7.25  7.35  7.45  7.55  7.65  7.75  7.85  7.95  8.1  8.2  8.3  8.4  8.5  8.6  8.75  8.85  8.95  9.05

FOR EDGE LIFT   0.01 ,   OPTIC DIAMETERS   8.5 - 9.5 ,   ZONAL CURVATURES ARE
 7.1  7.2  7.3  7.4  7.5  7.65  7.75  7.85  7.95  8.05  8.15  8.25  8.4  8.5  8.6  8.7  8.8  8.9  9.05

FOR EDGE LIFT   0.01 ,   OPTIC DIAMETERS   9 - 10 ,   ZONAL CURVATURES ARE
 7.1  7.2  7.3  7.4  7.5  7.6  7.7  7.8  7.95  8.05  8.15  8.25  8.35  8.45  8.55  8.7  8.8  8.9  9

FOR EDGE LIFT   0.01 ,   OPTIC DIAMETERS   9.5 - 10.5 ,   ZONAL CURVATURES ARE
 7.05  7.15  7.3  7.4  7.5  7.6  7.7  7.8  7.9  8  8.1  8.25  8.35  8.45  8.55  8.65  8.75  8.85  9

FOR EDGE LIFT   0.01 ,   OPTIC DIAMETERS   10 - 11 ,   ZONAL CURVATURES ARE
 7.05  7.15  7.25  7.35  7.45  7.6  7.7  7.8  7.9  8  8.1  8.2  8.3  8.45  8.55  8.65  8.75  8.85  8.95

FOR EDGE LIFT   0.01 ,   OPTIC DIAMETERS   10.5 - 11.5 ,   ZONAL CURVATURES ARE
 7.05  7.15  7.25  7.35  7.45  7.55  7.65  7.8  7.9  8  8.1  8.2  8.3  8.4  8.5  8.6  8.75  8.85  8.95

FOR EDGE LIFT   0.01 ,   OPTIC DIAMETERS   11 - 12 ,   ZONAL CURVATURES ARE
 7.05  7.15  7.25  7.35  7.45  7.55  7.65  7.75  7.85  7.95  8.1  8.2  8.3  8.4  8.5  8.6  8.7  8.8  8.9
```

```
FOR EDGE LIFT   0.02 ,   OPTIC DIAMETERS   6 - 7 ,   ZONAL CURVATURES ARE
 7.45  7.6  7.7  7.8  7.95  8.05  8.2  8.3  8.4  8.55  8.65  8.8  8.9  9.05  9.15  9.3  9.4  9.55  9.65

FOR EDGE LIFT   0.02 ,   OPTIC DIAMETERS   6.5 - 7.5 ,   ZONAL CURVATURES ARE
 7.4  7.5  7.65  7.75  7.85  8  8.1  8.2  8.35  8.45  8.6  8.7  8.8  8.95  9.05  9.2  9.3  9.45  9.55

FOR EDGE LIFT   0.02 ,   OPTIC DIAMETERS   7 - 8 ,   ZONAL CURVATURES ARE
 7.35  7.45  7.55  7.7  7.8  7.9  8.05  8.15  8.25  8.4  8.5  8.65  8.75  8.85  9  9.1  9.25  9.35  9.45

FOR EDGE LIFT   0.02 ,   OPTIC DIAMETERS   7.5 - 8.5 ,   ZONAL CURVATURES ARE
 7.3  7.4  7.5  7.65  7.75  7.85  8  8.1  8.2  8.35  8.45  8.55  8.7  8.8  8.9  9.05  9.15  9.3  9.4

FOR EDGE LIFT   0.02 ,   OPTIC DIAMETERS   8 - 9 ,   ZONAL CURVATURES ARE
 7.25  7.35  7.45  7.6  7.7  7.8  7.95  8.05  8.15  8.3  8.4  8.5  8.65  8.75  8.85  9  9.1  9.2  9.35

FOR EDGE LIFT   0.02 ,   OPTIC DIAMETERS   8.5 - 9.5 ,   ZONAL CURVATURES ARE
 7.2  7.3  7.45  7.55  7.65  7.75  7.9  8  8.1  8.25  8.35  8.45  8.55  8.7  8.8  8.9  9.05  9.15  9.25

FOR EDGE LIFT   0.02 ,   OPTIC DIAMETERS   9 - 10 ,   ZONAL CURVATURES ARE
 7.15  7.3  7.4  7.5  7.6  7.75  7.85  7.95  8.05  8.2  8.3  8.4  8.55  8.65  8.75  8.85  9  9.1  9.2

FOR EDGE LIFT   0.02 ,   OPTIC DIAMETERS   9.5 - 10.5 ,   ZONAL CURVATURES ARE
 7.15  7.25  7.35  7.45  7.6  7.7  7.8  7.9  8.05  8.15  8.25  8.35  8.5  8.6  8.7  8.85  8.95  9.05  9.15

FOR EDGE LIFT   0.02 ,   OPTIC DIAMETERS   10 - 11 ,   ZONAL CURVATURES ARE
 7.1  7.2  7.35  7.45  7.55  7.65  7.75  7.9  8  8.1  8.2  8.35  8.45  8.55  8.65  8.8  8.9  9  9.1

FOR EDGE LIFT   0.02 ,   OPTIC DIAMETERS   10.5 - 11.5 ,   ZONAL CURVATURES ARE
 7.1  7.2  7.3  7.4  7.5  7.65  7.75  7.85  7.95  8.1  8.2  8.3  8.4  8.5  8.65  8.75  8.85  8.95  9.1

FOR EDGE LIFT   0.02 ,   OPTIC DIAMETERS   11 - 12 ,   ZONAL CURVATURES ARE
 7.05  7.15  7.3  7.4  7.5  7.6  7.7  7.85  7.95  8.05  8.15  8.25  8.4  8.5  8.6  8.7  8.8  8.95  9.05
```

FOR EDGE LIFT 0.03 , OPTIC DIAMETERS 6 - 7 , ZONAL CURVATURES ARE

7.7 7.85 8 8.1 8.25 8.4 8.5 8.65 8.8 8.9 9.05 9.2 9.35 9.45 9.6 9.75 9.9 10 10.15

FOR EDGE LIFT 0.03 , OPTIC DIAMETERS 6.5 - 7.5 , ZONAL CURVATURES ARE

7.6 7.75 7.85 8 8.15 8.25 8.4 8.5 8.65 8.8 8.9 9.05 9.2 9.3 9.45 9.6 9.75 9.85 10

FOR EDGE LIFT 0.03 , OPTIC DIAMETERS 7 - 8 , ZONAL CURVATURES ARE

7.55 7.65 7.8 7.9 8.05 8.15 8.3 8.4 8.55 8.65 8.8 8.95 9.05 9.2 9.35 9.45 9.6 9.75 9.85

FOR EDGE LIFT 0.03 , OPTIC DIAMETERS 7.5 - 8.5 , ZONAL CURVATURES ARE

7.45 7.55 7.7 7.8 7.95 8.05 8.2 8.3 8.45 8.6 8.7 8.85 8.95 9.1 9.2 9.35 9.5 9.6 9.75

FOR EDGE LIFT 0.03 , OPTIC DIAMETERS 8 - 9 , ZONAL CURVATURES ARE

7.4 7.5 7.6 7.75 7.85 8 8.1 8.25 8.35 8.5 8.6 3.75 8.85 9 9.1 9.25 9.4 9.5 9.65

FOR EDGE LIFT 0.03 , OPTIC DIAMETERS 8.5 - 9.5 , ZONAL CURVATURES ARE

7.3 7.45 7.55 7.7 7.8 7.9 8.05 8.15 8.3 8.4 8.55 8.65 8.8 8.9 9.05 9.15 9.3 9.4 9.55

FOR EDGE LIFT 0.03 , OPTIC DIAMETERS 9 - 10 , ZONAL CURVATURES ARE

7.25 7.4 7.5 7.6 7.75 7.85 8 8.1 8.2 8.35 8.45 8.6 8.7 8.85 8.95 9.1 9.2 9.35 9.45

FOR EDGE LIFT 0.03 , OPTIC DIAMETERS 9.5 - 10.5 , ZONAL CURVATURES ARE

7.2 7.35 7.45 7.55 7.7 7.8 7.9 8.05 8.15 8.3 8.4 8.5 8.65 8.75 8.9 9 9.15 9.25 9.35

FOR EDGE LIFT 0.03 , OPTIC DIAMETERS 10 - 11 , ZONAL CURVATURES ARE

7.15 7.3 7.4 7.5 7.65 7.75 7.85 8 8.1 8.2 8.35 8.45 8.6 8.7 8.8 8.95 9.05 9.2 9.3

FOR EDGE LIFT 0.03 , OPTIC DIAMETERS 10.5 - 11.5 , ZONAL CURVATURES ARE

7.15 7.25 7.35 7.45 7.6 7.7 7.8 7.95 8.05 8.15 8.3 8.4 8.5 8.65 8.75 8.9 9 9.1 9.25

FOR EDGE LIFT 0.03 , OPTIC DIAMETERS 11 - 12 , ZONAL CURVATURES ARE

7.1 7.2 7.3 7.45 7.55 7.65 7.8 7.9 8 8.1 8.25 8.35 8.45 8.6 8.7 8.85 8.95 9.05 9.2

```
FOR EDGE LIFT   0.04 ,   OPTIC DIAMETERS   6  -  7 ,    ZONAL CURVATURES ARE
 8  8.15  8.3  8.45  8.6  8.75  8.9  9.05  9.2  9.35  9.5  9.65  9.8  9.95  10.1  10.25  10.4  10.6  10.75

FOR EDGE LIFT   0.04 ,   OPTIC DIAMETERS   6.5  -  7.5 ,    ZONAL CURVATURES ARE
 7.85  8  8.15  8.3  8.4  8.55  8.7  8.85  9  9.15  9.3  9.45  9.6  9.75  9.9  10.05  10.2  10.35  10.5

FOR EDGE LIFT   0.04 ,   OPTIC DIAMETERS   7  -  8 ,    ZONAL CURVATURES ARE
 7.75  7.85  8  8.15  8.3  8.4  8.55  8.7  8.85  9  9.1  9.25  9.4  9.55  9.7  9.85  10  10.15  10.3

FOR EDGE LIFT   0.04 ,   OPTIC DIAMETERS   7.5  -  8.5 ,    ZONAL CURVATURES ARE
 7.6  7.75  7.9  8  8.15  8.3  8.45  8.55  8.7  8.85  9  9.1  9.25  9.4  9.55  9.7  9.85  9.95  10.1

FOR EDGE LIFT   0.04 ,   OPTIC DIAMETERS   8  -  9 ,    ZONAL CURVATURES ARE
 7.5  7.65  7.8  7.9  8.05  8.2  8.3  8.45  8.6  8.7  8.85  9  9.15  9.25  9.4  9.55  9.7  9.8  9.95

FOR EDGE LIFT   0.04 ,   OPTIC DIAMETERS   8.5  -  9.5 ,    ZONAL CURVATURES ARE
 7.45  7.55  7.7  7.8  7.95  8.1  8.2  8.35  8.45  8.6  8.75  8.85  9  9.15  9.3  9.4  9.55  9.7  9.85

FOR EDGE LIFT   0.04 ,   OPTIC DIAMETERS   9  -  10 ,    ZONAL CURVATURES ARE
 7.35  7.5  7.6  7.75  7.85  8  8.1  8.25  8.4  8.5  8.65  8.75  8.9  9.05  9.15  9.3  9.45  9.55  9.7

FOR EDGE LIFT   0.04 ,   OPTIC DIAMETERS   9.5  -  10.5 ,    ZONAL CURVATURES ARE
 7.3  7.4  7.55  7.65  7.8  7.9  8.05  8.15  8.3  8.4  8.55  8.7  8.8  8.95  9.05  9.2  9.35  9.45  9.6

FOR EDGE LIFT   0.04 ,   OPTIC DIAMETERS   10  -  11 ,    ZONAL CURVATURES ARE
 7.25  7.35  7.5  7.6  7.7  7.85  7.95  8.1  8.2  8.35  8.45  8.6  8.7  8.85  9  9.1  9.25  9.35  9.5

FOR EDGE LIFT   0.04 ,   OPTIC DIAMETERS   10.5  -  11.5 ,    ZONAL CURVATURES ARE
 7.2  7.3  7.4  7.55  7.65  7.8  7.9  8  8.15  8.25  8.4  8.5  8.65  8.75  8.9  9  9.15  9.3  9.4

FOR EDGE LIFT   0.04 ,   OPTIC DIAMETERS   11  -  12 ,    ZONAL CURVATURES ARE
 7.15  7.25  7.35  7.5  7.6  7.7  7.85  7.95  8.1  8.2  8.35  8.45  8.55  8.7  8.8  8.95  9.05  9.2  9.3
```

FOR EDGE LIFT 0.05 , OPTIC DIAMETERS 6 - 7 , ZONAL CURVATURES ARE

8.3 8.5 8.65 8.8 8.95 9.15 9.3 9.45 9.65 9.8 9.95 10.15 10.3 10.5 10.65 10.85 11.05 11.2 11.4

FOR EDGE LIFT 0.05 , OPTIC DIAMETERS 6.5 - 7.5 , ZONAL CURVATURES ARE

8.1 8.25 8.45 8.6 8.75 8.9 9.05 9.2 9.4 9.55 9.7 9.85 10.05 10.2 10.35 10.55 10.7 10.9 11.05

FOR EDGE LIFT 0.05 , OPTIC DIAMETERS 7 - 8 , ZONAL CURVATURES ARE

7.95 8.1 8.25 8.4 8.55 8.7 8.85 9 9.15 9.3 9.5 9.65 9.8 9.95 10.1 10.3 10.45 10.6 10.8

FOR EDGE LIFT 0.05 , OPTIC DIAMETERS 7.5 - 8.5 , ZONAL CURVATURES ARE

7.8 7.95 8.1 8.25 8.4 8.55 8.7 8.85 9 9.15 9.3 9.45 9.6 9.75 9.9 10.05 10.2 10.35 10.55

FOR EDGE LIFT 0.05 , OPTIC DIAMETERS 8 - 9 , ZONAL CURVATURES ARE

7.7 7.8 7.95 8.1 8.25 8.4 8.55 8.65 8.8 8.95 9.1 9.25 9.4 9.55 9.7 9.85 10 10.15 10.3

FOR EDGE LIFT 0.05 , OPTIC DIAMETERS 8.5 - 9.5 , ZONAL CURVATURES ARE

7.55 7.7 7.85 8 8.1 8.25 8.4 8.55 8.7 8.8 8.95 9.1 9.25 9.4 9.55 9.7 9.85 10 10.15

FOR EDGE LIFT 0.05 , OPTIC DIAMETERS 9 - 10 , ZONAL CURVATURES ARE

7.45 7.6 7.75 7.85 8 8.15 8.25 8.4 8.55 8.7 8.85 8.95 9.1 9.25 9.4 9.55 9.7 9.85 10

FOR EDGE LIFT 0.05 , OPTIC DIAMETERS 9.5 - 10.5 , ZONAL CURVATURES ARE

7.4 7.5 7.65 7.75 7.9 8.05 8.15 8.3 8.45 8.55 8.7 8.85 9 9.1 9.25 9.4 9.55 9.7 9.85

FOR EDGE LIFT 0.05 , OPTIC DIAMETERS 10 - 11 , ZONAL CURVATURES ARE

7.3 7.45 7.55 7.7 7.8 7.95 8.05 8.2 8.35 8.45 8.6 8.75 8.85 9 9.15 9.3 9.4 9.55 9.7

FOR EDGE LIFT 0.05 , OPTIC DIAMETERS 10.5 - 11.5 , ZONAL CURVATURES ARE

7.25 7.35 7.5 7.6 7.75 7.85 8 8.1 8.25 8.4 8.5 8.65 8.75 8.9 9.05 9.15 9.3 9.45 9.6

FOR EDGE LIFT 0.05 , OPTIC DIAMETERS 11 - 12 , ZONAL CURVATURES ARE

7.15 7.3 7.4 7.55 7.65 7.8 7.9 8.05 8.15 8.3 8.4 8.55 8.7 8.8 8.95 9.05 9.2 9.35 9.45

```
FOR EDGE LIFT   6.00000E-2 ,   OPTIC DIAMETERS   6  -  7 ,   ZONAL CURVATURES ARE
 8.65  8.85  9  9.2  9.4  9.55  9.75  9.95  10.15  10.35  10.5  10.7  10.9  11.1  11.3  11.5  11.75  11.95  12.15

FOR EDGE LIFT   6.00000E-2 ,   OPTIC DIAMETERS   6.5  -  7.5 ,   ZONAL CURVATURES ARE
 8.4  8.6  8.75  8.9  9.1  9.25  9.45  9.6  9.8  10  10.15  10.35  10.55  10.7  10.9  11.1  11.3  11.5  11.7

FOR EDGE LIFT   6.00000E-2 ,   OPTIC DIAMETERS   7  -  8 ,   ZONAL CURVATURES ARE
 8.2  8.35  8.5  8.7  8.85  9  9.2  9.35  9.5  9.7  9.85  10.05  10.2  10.4  10.6  10.75  10.95  11.15  11.3

FOR EDGE LIFT   6.00000E-2 ,   OPTIC DIAMETERS   7.5  -  8.5 ,   ZONAL CURVATURES ARE
 8  8.15  8.3  8.45  8.65  8.8  8.95  9.1  9.3  9.45  9.6  9.8  9.95  10.1  10.3  10.45  10.65  10.8  11

FOR EDGE LIFT   6.00000E-2 ,   OPTIC DIAMETERS   8  -  9 ,   ZONAL CURVATURES ARE
 7.85  8  8.15  8.3  8.45  8.6  8.75  8.9  9.05  9.25  9.4  9.55  9.7  9.9  10.05  10.2  10.4  10.55  10.7

FOR EDGE LIFT   6.00000E-2 ,   OPTIC DIAMETERS   8.5  -  9.5 ,   ZONAL CURVATURES ARE
 7.7  7.85  8  8.15  8.3  8.45  8.6  8.75  8.9  9.05  9.2  9.35  9.5  9.65  9.85  10  10.15  10.3  10.5

FOR EDGE LIFT   6.00000E-2 ,   OPTIC DIAMETERS   9  -  10 ,   ZONAL CURVATURES ARE
 7.6  7.7  7.85  8  8.15  8.3  8.45  8.6  8.75  8.9  9.05  9.2  9.35  9.5  9.65  9.8  9.95  10.1  10.25

FOR EDGE LIFT   6.00000E-2 ,   OPTIC DIAMETERS   9.5  -  10.5 ,   ZONAL CURVATURES ARE
 7.45  7.6  7.75  7.9  8  8.15  8.3  8.45  8.6  8.75  8.9  9.05  9.2  9.35  9.5  9.65  9.8  9.95  10.1

FOR EDGE LIFT   6.00000E-2 ,   OPTIC DIAMETERS   10  -  11 ,   ZONAL CURVATURES ARE
 7.35  7.5  7.65  7.75  7.9  8.05  8.2  8.3  8.45  8.6  8.75  8.9  9.05  9.2  9.35  9.45  9.6  9.75  9.9

FOR EDGE LIFT   6.00000E-2 ,   OPTIC DIAMETERS   10.5  -  11.5 ,   ZONAL CURVATURES ARE
 7.3  7.4  7.55  7.7  7.8  7.95  8.1  8.2  8.35  8.5  8.65  8.75  8.9  9.05  9.2  9.35  9.5  9.6  9.75

FOR EDGE LIFT   6.00000E-2 ,   OPTIC DIAMETERS   11  -  12 ,   ZONAL CURVATURES ARE
 7.2  7.35  7.45  7.6  7.7  7.85  8  8.1  8.25  8.4  8.5  8.65  8.8  8.95  9.05  9.2  9.35  9.5  9.65
```

```
FOR EDGE LIFT   0.07 ,   OPTIC DIAMETERS   6 - 7 ,   ZONAL CURVATURES ARE
 9.05  9.25  9.45  9.65  9.85  10.05  10.3  10.5  10.7  10.95  11.15  11.35  11.6  11.85  12.05  12.3  12.55  12.8  13.05

FOR EDGE LIFT   0.07 ,   OPTIC DIAMETERS   6.5 - 7.5 ,   ZONAL CURVATURES ARE
 8.75  8.9  9.1  9.3  9.5  9.7  9.85  10.05  10.25  10.5  10.7  10.9  11.1  11.3  11.55  11.75  11.95  12.2  12.4

FOR EDGE LIFT   0.07 ,   OPTIC DIAMETERS   7 - 8 ,   ZONAL CURVATURES ARE
 8.45  8.65  8.8  9  9.15  9.35  9.55  9.75  9.9  10.1  10.3  10.5  10.7  10.9  11.1  11.3  11.5  11.7  11.95

FOR EDGE LIFT   0.07 ,   OPTIC DIAMETERS   7.5 - 8.5 ,   ZONAL CURVATURES ARE
 8.2  8.4  8.55  8.75  8.9  9.1  9.25  9.45  9.6  9.8  10  10.15  10.35  10.55  10.75  10.9  11.1  11.3  11.5

FOR EDGE LIFT   0.07 ,   OPTIC DIAMETERS   8 - 9 ,   ZONAL CURVATURES ARE
 8  8.2  8.35  8.5  8.65  8.85  9  9.2  9.35  9.55  9.7  9.9  10.05  10.25  10.4  10.6  10.8  10.95  11.15

FOR EDGE LIFT   0.07 ,   OPTIC DIAMETERS   8.5 - 9.5 ,   ZONAL CURVATURES ARE
 7.85  8  8.15  8.3  8.5  8.65  8.8  8.95  9.15  9.3  9.45  9.65  9.8  9.95  10.15  10.3  10.5  10.7  10.85

FOR EDGE LIFT   0.07 ,   OPTIC DIAMETERS   9 - 10 ,   ZONAL CURVATURES ARE
 7.7  7.85  8  8.15  8.3  8.45  8.6  8.75  8.95  9.1  9.25  9.4  9.6  9.75  9.9  10.1  10.25  10.4  10.6

FOR EDGE LIFT   0.07 ,   OPTIC DIAMETERS   9.5 - 10.5 ,   ZONAL CURVATURES ARE
 7.55  7.7  7.85  8  8.15  8.3  8.45  8.6  8.75  8.9  9.05  9.2  9.4  9.55  9.7  9.85  10.05  10.2  10.35

FOR EDGE LIFT   0.07 ,   OPTIC DIAMETERS   10 - 11 ,   ZONAL CURVATURES ARE
 7.45  7.6  7.7  7.85  8  8.15  8.3  8.45  8.6  8.75  8.9  9.05  9.2  9.35  9.5  9.7  9.85  10  10.15

FOR EDGE LIFT   0.07 ,   OPTIC DIAMETERS   10.5 - 11.5 ,   ZONAL CURVATURES ARE
 7.35  7.45  7.6  7.75  7.9  8.05  8.15  8.3  8.45  8.6  8.75  8.9  9.05  9.2  9.35  9.5  9.65  9.8  9.95

FOR EDGE LIFT   0.07 ,   OPTIC DIAMETERS   11 - 12 ,   ZONAL CURVATURES ARE
 7.25  7.4  7.5  7.65  7.8  7.9  8.05  8.2  8.35  8.5  8.6  8.75  8.9  9.05  9.2  9.35  9.5  9.65  9.8
```

```
FOR EDGE LIFT   0.08 ,   OPTIC DIAMETERS   6 - 7 ,   ZONAL CURVATURES ARE
 9.5  9.7  9.95  10.15  10.4  10.65  10.85  11.1  11.35  11.6  11.85  12.1  12.4  12.65  12.95  13.2  13.5  13.75  14.05

FOR EDGE LIFT   0.08 ,   OPTIC DIAMETERS   6.5 - 7.5 ,   ZONAL CURVATURES ARE
 9.1  9.3  9.5  9.7  9.9  10.15  10.35  10.6  10.8  11.05  11.25  11.5  11.75  12  12.25  12.5  12.75  13  13.25

FOR EDGE LIFT   0.08 ,   OPTIC DIAMETERS   7 - 8 ,   ZONAL CURVATURES ARE
 8.75  8.95  9.15  9.35  9.55  9.75  9.95  10.15  10.35  10.55  10.8  11  11.2  11.45  11.7  11.9  12.15  12.4  12.6

FOR EDGE LIFT   0.08 ,   OPTIC DIAMETERS   7.5 - 8.5 ,   ZONAL CURVATURES ARE
 8.45  8.65  8.8  9  9.2  9.4  9.6  9.8  10  10.2  10.4  10.6  10.8  11  11.2  11.45  11.65  11.85  12.1

FOR EDGE LIFT   0.08 ,   OPTIC DIAMETERS   8 - 9 ,   ZONAL CURVATURES ARE
 8.2  8.4  8.55  8.75  8.9  9.1  9.3  9.45  9.65  9.85  10.05  10.25  10.45  10.6  10.85  11.05  11.25  11.45  11.65

FOR EDGE LIFT   0.08 ,   OPTIC DIAMETERS   8.5 - 9.5 ,   ZONAL CURVATURES ARE
 8  8.15  8.35  8.5  8.7  8.85  9  9.2  9.4  9.55  9.75  9.95  10.1  10.3  10.5  10.7  10.9  11.1  11.25

FOR EDGE LIFT   0.08 ,   OPTIC DIAMETERS   9 - 10 ,   ZONAL CURVATURES ARE
 7.8  8  8.15  8.3  8.45  8.65  8.8  8.95  9.15  9.3  9.5  9.65  9.85  10  10.2  10.4  10.55  10.75  10.95

FOR EDGE LIFT   0.08 ,   OPTIC DIAMETERS   9.5 - 10.5 ,   ZONAL CURVATURES ARE
 7.65  7.8  7.95  8.1  8.3  8.45  8.6  8.75  8.95  9.1  9.25  9.45  9.6  9.8  9.95  10.15  10.3  10.5  10.65

FOR EDGE LIFT   0.08 ,   OPTIC DIAMETERS   10 - 11 ,   ZONAL CURVATURES ARE
 7.5  7.65  7.8  7.95  8.1  8.25  8.45  8.6  8.75  8.9  9.05  9.25  9.4  9.55  9.75  9.9  10.05  10.25  10.4

FOR EDGE LIFT   0.08 ,   OPTIC DIAMETERS   10.5 - 11.5 ,   ZONAL CURVATURES ARE
 7.4  7.55  7.7  7.85  7.95  8.1  8.25  8.45  8.6  8.75  8.9  9.05  9.2  9.35  9.55  9.7  9.85  10  10.2

FOR EDGE LIFT   0.08 ,   OPTIC DIAMETERS   11 - 12 ,   ZONAL CURVATURES ARE
 7.3  7.45  7.55  7.7  7.85  8  8.15  8.3  8.45  8.6  8.75  8.9  9.05  9.2  9.35  9.5  9.65  9.85  10
```

```
FOR EDGE LIFT   0.09 ,   OPTIC DIAMETERS   6 - 7 ,   ZONAL CURVATURES ARE
 9.95  10.2  10.5  10.75  11  11.25  11.55  11.8  12.1  12.4  12.7  13  13.3  13.6  13.95  14.25  14.6  14.95  15.3

FOR EDGE LIFT   0.09 ,   OPTIC DIAMETERS   6.5 - 7.5 ,   ZONAL CURVATURES ARE
 9.45  9.7  9.95  10.15  10.4  10.65  10.9  11.15  11.4  11.65  11.95  12.2  12.5  12.75  13.05  13.35  13.65  13.95  14.25

FOR EDGE LIFT   0.09 ,   OPTIC DIAMETERS   7 - 8 ,   ZONAL CURVATURES ARE
 9.05  9.25  9.5  9.7  9.9  10.15  10.35  10.6  10.85  11.1  11.3  11.55  11.8  12.05  12.35  12.6  12.85  13.15  13.4

FOR EDGE LIFT   0.09 ,   OPTIC DIAMETERS   7.5 - 8.5 ,   ZONAL CURVATURES ARE
 8.7  8.9  9.1  9.3  9.5  9.75  9.95  10.15  10.4  10.6  10.8  11.05  11.3  11.5  11.75  12  12.25  12.5  12.75

FOR EDGE LIFT   0.09 ,   OPTIC DIAMETERS   8 - 9 ,   ZONAL CURVATURES ARE
 8.4  8.6  8.8  9  9.2  9.4  9.6  9.3  10  10.2  10.4  10.6  10.85  11.05  11.3  11.5  11.75  11.95  12.2

FOR EDGE LIFT   0.09 ,   OPTIC DIAMETERS   8.5 - 9.5 ,   ZONAL CURVATURES ARE
 8.15  8.35  8.55  8.7  8.9  9.1  9.25  9.45  9.65  9.85  10.05  10.25  10.45  10.65  10.85  11.1  11.3  11.5  11.75

FOR EDGE LIFT   0.09 ,   OPTIC DIAMETERS   9 - 10 ,   ZONAL CURVATURES ARE
 7.95  8.1  8.3  8.45  8.65  8.8  9  9.2  9.35  9.55  9.75  9.95  10.15  10.3  10.5  10.7  10.9  11.15  11.35

FOR EDGE LIFT   0.09 ,   OPTIC DIAMETERS   9.5 - 10.5 ,   ZONAL CURVATURES ARE
 7.75  7.9  8.1  8.25  8.4  8.6  8.75  8.95  9.1  9.3  9.45  9.65  9.85  10.05  10.2  10.4  10.6  10.8  11

FOR EDGE LIFT   0.09 ,   OPTIC DIAMETERS   10 - 11 ,   ZONAL CURVATURES ARE
 7.6  7.75  7.9  8.05  8.25  8.4  8.55  8.75  8.9  9.05  9.25  9.4  9.6  9.75  9.95  10.15  10.3  10.5  10.7

FOR EDGE LIFT   0.09 ,   OPTIC DIAMETERS   10.5 - 11.5 ,   ZONAL CURVATURES ARE
 7.45  7.6  7.75  7.9  8.05  8.2  8.4  8.55  8.7  8.85  9.05  9.2  9.35  9.55  9.7  9.9  10.05  10.25  10.4

FOR EDGE LIFT   0.09 ,   OPTIC DIAMETERS   11 - 12 ,   ZONAL CURVATURES ARE
 7.35  7.5  7.6  7.75  7.9  8.05  8.2  8.35  8.55  8.7  8.85  9  9.15  9.35  9.5  9.65  9.85  10  10.2
```

FOR EDGE LIFT 0.1 , OPTIC DIAMETERS 6 - 7 , ZONAL CURVATURES ARE

10.55 10.8 11.1 11.4 11.7 12 12.3 12.65 13 13.3 13.65 14 14.4 14.75 15.15 15.55 15.95 16.35 16.75

FOR EDGE LIFT 0.1 , OPTIC DIAMETERS 6.5 - 7.5 , ZONAL CURVATURES ARE

9.9 10.15 10.4 10.7 10.95 11.25 11.5 11.8 12.1 12.4 12.7 13 13.3 13.65 14 14.3 14.65 15 15.4

FOR EDGE LIFT 0.1 , OPTIC DIAMETERS 7 - 8 , ZONAL CURVATURES ARE

9.4 9.65 9.85 10.1 10.35 10.6 10.85 11.15 11.4 11.65 11.95 12.2 12.5 12.8 13.1 13.4 13.7 14 14.3

FOR EDGE LIFT 0.1 , OPTIC DIAMETERS 7.5 - 8.5 , ZONAL CURVATURES ARE

9 9.2 9.4 9.65 9.9 10.1 10.35 10.6 10.8 11.05 11.3 11.55 11.85 12.1 12.35 12.65 12.9 13.2 13.5

FOR EDGE LIFT 0.1 , OPTIC DIAMETERS 8 - 9 , ZONAL CURVATURES ARE

8.65 8.85 9.05 9.25 9.45 9.7 9.9 10.15 10.35 10.6 10.8 11.05 11.3 11.55 11.8 12.05 12.3 12.55 12.8

FOR EDGE LIFT 0.1 , OPTIC DIAMETERS 8.5 - 9.5 , ZONAL CURVATURES ARE

8.35 8.55 8.75 8.95 9.15 9.35 9.55 9.75 9.95 10.15 10.4 10.6 10.85 11.05 11.3 11.5 11.75 12 12.25

FOR EDGE LIFT 0.1 , OPTIC DIAMETERS 9 - 10 , ZONAL CURVATURES ARE

8.1 8.25 8.45 8.65 8.85 9 9.2 9.4 9.6 9.8 10 10.25 10.45 10.65 10.85 11.1 11.3 11.55 11.75

FOR EDGE LIFT 0.1 , OPTIC DIAMETERS 9.5 - 10.5 , ZONAL CURVATURES ARE

7.85 8.05 8.2 8.4 8.6 8.75 8.95 9.15 9.3 9.5 9.7 9.9 10.1 10.3 10.5 10.7 10.9 11.15 11.35

FOR EDGE LIFT 0.1 , OPTIC DIAMETERS 10 - 11 , ZONAL CURVATURES ARE

7.7 7.85 8 8.2 8.35 8.55 8.7 8.9 9.05 9.25 9.45 9.6 9.8 10 10.2 10.4 10.6 10.8 11

FOR EDGE LIFT 0.1 , OPTIC DIAMETERS 10.5 - 11.5 , ZONAL CURVATURES ARE

7.5 7.7 7.85 8 8.15 8.3 8.5 8.65 8.85 9 9.2 9.35 9.55 9.75 9.9 10.1 10.3 10.5 10.65

FOR EDGE LIFT 0.1 , OPTIC DIAMETERS 11 - 12 , ZONAL CURVATURES ARE

7.4 7.55 7.7 7.85 8 8.15 8.3 8.45 8.65 8.8 8.95 9.15 9.3 9.5 9.65 9.85 10.05 10.2 10.4

FOR EDGE LIFT 0.11 , OPTIC DIAMETERS 6 - 7 , ZONAL CURVATURES ARE

11.15 11.5 11.8 12.15 12.5 12.85 13.25 13.6 14 14.4 14.8 15.25 15.65 16.1 16.6 17.05 17.55 18.05 18.6

FOR EDGE LIFT 0.11 , OPTIC DIAMETERS 6.5 - 7.5 , ZONAL CURVATURES ARE

10.4 10.65 10.95 11.25 11.55 11.9 12.2 12.55 12.9 13.2 13.6 13.95 14.3 14.7 15.1 15.5 15.9 16.3 16.75

FOR EDGE LIFT 0.11 , OPTIC DIAMETERS 7 - 8 , ZONAL CURVATURES ARE

9.8 10.05 10.3 10.6 10.85 11.15 11.4 11.7 12 12.3 12.65 12.95 13.25 13.6 13.95 14.3 14.65 15 15.4

FOR EDGE LIFT 0.11 , OPTIC DIAMETERS 7.5 - 8.5 , ZONAL CURVATURES ARE

9.3 9.55 9.75 10 10.25 10.5 10.8 11.05 11.3 11.6 11.85 12.15 12.45 12.75 13.05 13.35 13.7 14 14.35

FOR EDGE LIFT 0.11 , OPTIC DIAMETERS 8 - 9 , ZONAL CURVATURES ARE

8.9 9.1 9.35 9.55 9.8 10 10.25 10.5 10.75 11 11.25 11.5 11.8 12.05 12.35 12.6 12.9 13.2 13.5

FOR EDGE LIFT 0.11 , OPTIC DIAMETERS 8.5 - 9.5 , ZONAL CURVATURES ARE

8.55 8.75 8.95 9.15 9.4 9.6 9.8 10.05 10.3 10.5 10.75 11 11.25 11.5 11.75 12 12.25 12.55 12.8

FOR EDGE LIFT 0.11 , OPTIC DIAMETERS 9 - 10 , ZONAL CURVATURES ARE

8.25 8.45 8.65 8.85 9.05 9.25 9.45 9.65 9.9 10.1 10.3 10.55 10.75 11 11.25 11.5 11.75 12 12.25

FOR EDGE LIFT 0.11 , OPTIC DIAMETERS 9.5 - 10.5 , ZONAL CURVATURES ARE

8 8.15 8.35 8.55 8.75 8.95 9.15 9.35 9.55 9.75 9.95 10.15 10.4 10.6 10.8 11.05 11.25 11.5 11.75

FOR EDGE LIFT 0.11 , OPTIC DIAMETERS 10 - 11 , ZONAL CURVATURES ARE

7.75 7.95 8.1 8.3 8.5 8.65 8.85 9.05 9.25 9.45 9.65 9.85 10.05 10.25 10.45 10.65 10.85 11.1 11.3

FOR EDGE LIFT 0.11 , OPTIC DIAMETERS 10.5 - 11.5 , ZONAL CURVATURES ARE

7.6 7.75 7.9 8.1 8.25 8.45 8.6 8.8 8.95 9.15 9.35 9.55 9.75 9.95 10.1 10.35 10.55 10.75 10.95

FOR EDGE LIFT 0.11 , OPTIC DIAMETERS 11 - 12 , ZONAL CURVATURES ARE

7.4 7.6 7.75 7.9 8.05 8.25 8.4 8.55 8.75 8.9 9.1 9.3 9.45 9.65 9.85 10.05 10.25 10.4 10.6

```
FOR EDGE LIFT   0.12 ,   OPTIC DIAMETERS   6  -  7 ,   ZONAL CURVATURES ARE
 11.85  12.25  12.65  13.05  13.45  13.85  14.3  14.75  15.2  15.7  16.2  16.7  17.25  17.8  18.35  18.95  19.55  20.2  20.85

FOR EDGE LIFT   0.12 ,   OPTIC DIAMETERS   6.5  -  7.5 ,   ZONAL CURVATURES ARE
 10.95  11.25  11.6  11.95  12.3  12.65  13  13.4  13.8  14.2  14.6  15.05  15.45  15.9  16.4  16.85  17.35  17.9  18.4

FOR EDGE LIFT   0.12 ,   OPTIC DIAMETERS   7  -  8 ,   ZONAL CURVATURES ARE
 10.2  10.5  10.8  11.1  11.4  11.7  12.05  12.35  12.7  13.05  13.4  13.8  14.15  14.55  14.95  15.35  15.75  16.2  16.65

FOR EDGE LIFT   0.12 ,   OPTIC DIAMETERS   7.5  -  8.5 ,   ZONAL CURVATURES ARE
 9.6  9.9  10.15  10.4  10.7  11  11.25  11.55  11.85  12.2  12.5  12.8  13.15  13.5  13.85  14.2  14.55  14.95  15.3

FOR EDGE LIFT   0.12 ,   OPTIC DIAMETERS   8  -  9 ,   ZONAL CURVATURES ARE
 9.15  9.4  9.65  9.9  10.15  10.4  10.65  10.9  11.2  11.5  11.75  12.05  12.35  12.65  12.95  13.3  13.6  13.95  14.3

FOR EDGE LIFT   0.12 ,   OPTIC DIAMETERS   8.5  -  9.5 ,   ZONAL CURVATURES ARE
 8.75  8.95  9.2  9.4  9.65  9.9  10.15  10.4  10.65  10.9  11.15  11.4  11.7  11.95  12.25  12.55  12.85  13.15  13.45

FOR EDGE LIFT   0.12 ,   OPTIC DIAMETERS   9  -  10 ,   ZONAL CURVATURES ARE
 8.4  8.6  8.8  9.05  9.25  9.5  9.7  9.95  10.15  10.4  10.65  10.9  11.15  11.4  11.65  11.9  12.2  12.45  12.75

FOR EDGE LIFT   0.12 ,   OPTIC DIAMETERS   9.5  -  10.5 ,   ZONAL CURVATURES ARE
 8.1  8.3  8.5  8.7  8.9  9.1  9.35  9.55  9.75  10  10.2  10.45  10.7  10.9  11.15  11.4  11.65  11.9  12.15

FOR EDGE LIFT   0.12 ,   OPTIC DIAMETERS   10  -  11 ,   ZONAL CURVATURES ARE
 7.85  8.05  8.25  8.45  8.6  8.8  9  9.2  9.4  9.65  9.85  10.05  10.3  10.5  10.75  10.95  11.2  11.45  11.65

FOR EDGE LIFT   0.12 ,   OPTIC DIAMETERS   10.5  -  11.5 ,   ZONAL CURVATURES ARE
 7.65  7.85  8  8.2  8.35  8.55  8.75  8.95  9.1  9.3  9.5  9.7  9.95  10.15  10.35  10.55  10.8  11  11.25

FOR EDGE LIFT   0.12 ,   OPTIC DIAMETERS   11  -  12 ,   ZONAL CURVATURES ARE
 7.45  7.65  7.8  7.95  8.15  8.3  8.5  8.7  8.85  9.05  9.25  9.45  9.65  9.85  10.05  10.25  10.45  10.65  10.85
```

FOR EDGE LIFT 0.13 , OPTIC DIAMETERS 6 - 7 , ZONAL CURVATURES ARE

12.7 13.15 13.6 14.05 14.55 15.05 15.55 16.1 16.7 17.25 17.9 18.5 19.2 19.85 20.6 21.35 22.15 22.95 23.85

FOR EDGE LIFT 0.13 , OPTIC DIAMETERS 6.5 - 7.5 , ZONAL CURVATURES ARE

11.55 11.9 12.3 12.7 13.1 13.5 13.95 14.4 14.85 15.35 15.8 16.35 16.85 17.4 17.95 18.55 19.15 19.8 20.45

FOR EDGE LIFT 0.13 , OPTIC DIAMETERS 7 - 8 , ZONAL CURVATURES ARE

10.7 11 11.35 11.65 12 12.4 12.75 13.15 13.5 13.9 14.35 14.75 15.2 15.65 16.1 16.6 17.1 17.6 18.15

FOR EDGE LIFT 0.13 , OPTIC DIAMETERS 7.5 - 8.5 , ZONAL CURVATURES ARE

10 10.3 10.55 10.85 11.2 11.5 11.8 12.15 12.5 12.85 13.2 13.6 13.95 14.35 14.75 15.15 15.6 16 16.45

FOR EDGE LIFT 0.13 , OPTIC DIAMETERS 8 - 9 , ZONAL CURVATURES ARE

9.45 9.7 9.95 10.25 10.5 10.8 11.1 11.4 11.7 12 12.3 12.65 13 13.3 13.7 14.05 14.4 14.8 15.15

FOR EDGE LIFT 0.13 , OPTIC DIAMETERS 8.5 - 9.5 , ZONAL CURVATURES ARE

8.95 9.2 9.45 9.7 9.95 10.2 10.5 10.75 11.05 11.3 11.6 11.9 12.2 12.5 12.8 13.15 13.45 13.8 14.15

FOR EDGE LIFT 0.13 , OPTIC DIAMETERS 9 - 10 , ZONAL CURVATURES ARE

8.6 8.8 9 9.25 9.5 9.75 10 10.2 10.5 10.75 11 11.25 11.55 11.85 12.1 12.4 12.7 13 13.3

FOR EDGE LIFT 0.13 , OPTIC DIAMETERS 9.5 - 10.5 , ZONAL CURVATURES ARE

8.25 8.45 8.65 8.9 9.1 9.3 9.55 9.8 10 10.25 10.5 10.75 11 11.25 11.55 11.8 12.05 12.35 12.65

FOR EDGE LIFT 0.13 , OPTIC DIAMETERS 10 - 11 , ZONAL CURVATURES ARE

7.95 8.15 8.35 8.55 8.75 8.95 9.2 9.4 9.6 9.85 10.05 10.3 10.55 10.8 11.05 11.3 11.55 11.8 12.05

FOR EDGE LIFT 0.13 , OPTIC DIAMETERS 10.5 - 11.5 , ZONAL CURVATURES ARE

7.75 7.9 8.1 8.3 8.45 8.65 8.85 9.05 9.3 9.5 9.7 9.9 10.15 10.35 10.6 10.85 11.05 11.3 11.55

FOR EDGE LIFT 0.13 , OPTIC DIAMETERS 11 - 12 , ZONAL CURVATURES ARE

7.5 7.7 7.85 8.05 8.25 8.4 8.6 8.8 9 9.2 9.4 9.6 9.8 10 10.25 10.45 10.65 10.9 11.1

FOR EDGE LIFT 0.14 , OPTIC DIAMETERS 6 - 7 , ZONAL CURVATURES ARE

13.65 14.2 14.7 15.3 15.85 16.5 17.1 17.8 18.5 19.2 20 20.8 21.65 22.55 23.45 24.45 25.5 26.65 27.8

FOR EDGE LIFT 0.14 , OPTIC DIAMETERS 6.5 - 7.5 , ZONAL CURVATURES ARE

12.25 12.7 13.1 13.6 14.05 14.55 15.05 15.55 16.1 16.7 17.3 17.9 18.55 19.2 19.9 20.65 21.4 22.2 23.05

FOR EDGE LIFT 0.14 , OPTIC DIAMETERS 7 - 8 , ZONAL CURVATURES ARE

11.2 11.55 11.95 12.35 12.75 13.15 13.55 14 14.45 14.9 15.4 15.9 16.4 16.95 17.5 18.1 18.7 19.3 19.95

FOR EDGE LIFT 0.14 , OPTIC DIAMETERS 7.5 - 8.5 , ZONAL CURVATURES ARE

10.4 10.7 11.05 11.35 11.7 12.1 12.45 12.8 13.2 13.6 14 14.45 14.85 15.3 15.8 16.25 16.75 17.25 17.8

FOR EDGE LIFT 0.14 , OPTIC DIAMETERS 8 - 9 , ZONAL CURVATURES ARE

9.75 10 10.3 10.6 10.9 11.25 11.55 11.9 12.25 12.6 12.95 13.3 13.7 14.1 14.5 14.9 15.3 15.75 16.2

FOR EDGE LIFT 0.14 , OPTIC DIAMETERS 8.5 - 9.5 , ZONAL CURVATURES ARE

9.2 9.45 9.75 10 10.3 10.55 10.85 11.15 11.45 11.75 12.1 12.4 12.75 13.1 13.45 13.8 14.2 14.55 14.95

FOR EDGE LIFT 0.14 , OPTIC DIAMETERS 9 - 10 , ZONAL CURVATURES ARE

8.75 9 9.25 9.5 9.75 10 10.25 10.55 10.8 11.1 11.4 11.7 12 12.3 12.6 12.95 13.3 13.6 13.95

FOR EDGE LIFT 0.14 , OPTIC DIAMETERS 9.5 - 10.5 , ZONAL CURVATURES ARE

8.4 8.6 8.85 9.05 9.3 9.55 9.8 10.05 10.3 10.55 10.8 11.1 11.35 11.65 11.95 12.25 12.55 12.85 13.15

FOR EDGE LIFT 0.14 , OPTIC DIAMETERS 10 - 11 , ZONAL CURVATURES ARE

8.05 8.3 8.5 8.7 8.9 9.15 9.35 9.6 9.85 10.1 10.3 10.55 10.85 11.1 11.35 11.65 11.9 12.2 12.45

FOR EDGE LIFT 0.14 , OPTIC DIAMETERS 10.5 - 11.5 , ZONAL CURVATURES ARE

7.8 8 8.2 8.4 8.6 8.8 9 9.25 9.45 9.65 9.9 10.15 10.35 10.6 10.85 11.1 11.35 11.65 11.9

FOR EDGE LIFT 0.14 , OPTIC DIAMETERS 11 - 12 , ZONAL CURVATURES ARE

7.6 7.75 7.95 8.1 8.3 8.5 8.7 8.9 9.1 9.35 9.55 9.75 10 10.2 10.45 10.65 10.9 11.15 11.4

```
FOR EDGE LIFT   0.15 ,   OPTIC DIAMETERS   6 - 7 ,    ZONAL CURVATURES ARE

 14.8  15.45  16.1  16.75  17.5  18.25  19  19.85  20.75  21.65  22.65  23.7  24.85  26.05  27.3  28.7  30.15  31.75  33.45

FOR EDGE LIFT   0.15 ,   OPTIC DIAMETERS   6.5 - 7.5 ,    ZONAL CURVATURES ARE

 13.05  13.55  14.05  14.6  15.15  15.75  16.35  16.95  17.65  18.35  19.05  19.8  20.6  21.45  22.35  23.25  24.25  25.3
 26.4

FOR EDGE LIFT   0.15 ,   OPTIC DIAMETERS   7 - 8 ,    ZONAL CURVATURES ARE

 11.8  12.2  12.65  13.1  13.55  14  14.5  15  15.55  16.1  16.65  17.25  17.85  18.5  19.2  19.9  20.65  21.4  22.2

FOR EDGE LIFT   0.15 ,   OPTIC DIAMETERS   7.5 - 8.5 ,    ZONAL CURVATURES ARE

 10.85  11.2  11.55  11.95  12.3  12.75  13.15  13.55  14  14.45  14.95  15.45  15.95  16.45  17  17.6  18.15  18.75  19.4

FOR EDGE LIFT   0.15 ,   OPTIC DIAMETERS   8 - 9 ,    ZONAL CURVATURES ARE

 10.1  10.4  10.7  11.05  11.4  11.75  12.1  12.45  12.85  13.25  13.65  14.05  14.5  14.95  15.4  15.9  16.35  16.9  17.4

FOR EDGE LIFT   0.15 ,   OPTIC DIAMETERS   8.5 - 9.5 ,    ZONAL CURVATURES ARE

 9.45  9.75  10.05  10.35  10.65  10.95  11.25  11.6  11.95  12.3  12.65  13  13.4  13.75  14.15  14.6  15  15.45  15.9

FOR EDGE LIFT   0.15 ,   OPTIC DIAMETERS   9 - 10 ,    ZONAL CURVATURES ARE

 8.95  9.2  9.5  9.75  10  10.3  10.6  10.9  11.2  11.5  11.85  12.15  12.5  12.85  13.2  13.55  13.9  14.3  14.7

FOR EDGE LIFT   0.15 ,   OPTIC DIAMETERS   9.5 - 10.5 ,    ZONAL CURVATURES ARE

 8.55  8.75  9  9.25  9.5  9.75  10.05  10.3  10.6  10.85  11.15  11.45  11.75  12.05  12.4  12.7  13.05  13.4  13.75

FOR EDGE LIFT   0.15 ,   OPTIC DIAMETERS   10 - 11 ,    ZONAL CURVATURES ARE

 8.2  8.4  8.6  8.85  9.1  9.3  9.55  9.8  10.05  10.35  10.6  10.85  11.15  11.4  11.7  12  12.3  12.6  12.95

FOR EDGE LIFT   0.15 ,   OPTIC DIAMETERS   10.5 - 11.5 ,    ZONAL CURVATURES ARE

 7.9  8.1  8.3  8.5  8.7  8.95  9.15  9.4  9.65  9.85  10.1  10.35  10.6  10.9  11.15  11.4  11.7  12  12.25

FOR EDGE LIFT   0.15 ,   OPTIC DIAMETERS   11 - 12 ,    ZONAL CURVATURES ARE

 7.65  7.8  8  8.2  8.4  8.6  8.8  9.05  9.25  9.5  9.7  9.95  10.2  10.4  10.65  10.9  11.15  11.45  11.7
```

Made in the USA
Monee, IL
13 September 2026

62978960R10096